AF774358

THE MEDICINE OF PLANTS

THE MEDICINE OF PLANTS
Healing, Nature, and What It Means to Be Human

Peter Jackson-Main

AEON

First published in 2026 by
Aeon Books

Copyright © 2026 by Peter Jackson-Main

The right of Peter Jackson-Main to be identified as the author of this work has been asserted in accordance with §§ 77 and 78 of the Copyright Design and Patents Act 1988.

All rights reserved. No part of this publication may be reproduced, stored in a retrieval system, or transmitted, in any form or by any means, electronic, mechanical, photocopying, recording, or otherwise, without the prior written permission of the publisher.

British Library Cataloguing in Publication Data

A C.I.P. for this book is available from the British Library

ISBN-13: 978-1-80152-248-9

Typeset by Medlar Publishing Solutions Pvt Ltd, India

www.aeonbooks.co.uk

CONTENTS

DEDICATION AND ACKNOWLEDGMENTS

This book is dedicated to those who have been most influential in developing my perception of the unseen worlds, and my skill in navigating them:

Ato Rinpoche
Pajé Tchydjo
Gerrie March

The following people distinguish themselves through their contributions to my work, my wellbeing, and my wisdom, in recent months during the writing of this book:

Anji Main, my beloved partner and co-creator,
without whom I would but scarcely be what I am.

Davyd Farrell, my spiritual brother and sparring partner,
who assisted me in developing an inclusive and
multi-levelled approach to plant medicine.

Ya'acov Darling-Khan, who reintroduced me to movement medicine just in time to rescue the last few chapters from exhaustion and stagnation.

Rafi, our Saluki, who is the embodiment of joy and mischief, and dog medicine generally.

Magic, our black cat, who willingly and enthusiastically embraces the job of protector for our household, in return of course for top quality food.

My eternal spirit, who has kept this peculiar and idiosyncratic flame alight on earth for 70 years at the time of writing.

The plant people, my allies and teachers, without whom none of this would be meaningful, including but not limited to *Achillea millefolium, Angelica archangelica, Artemisia absinthium, Artemisia vulgaris, Astragalus membranaceus, Bannisteriopsis caapi, Berberis vulgaris, Capsicum minimum, Crataegus* spp., *Echinacea* spp., *Eleutherococcus senticosus, Equisetum arvense, Filipendula ulmaria, Hypericum perforatum, Nicotiana tabacum, Picea abies, Plantago* spp., *Psychotria viridis, Sambucus nigra, Taraxacum officinale, Taxus baccata, Urtica dioica*—and with apologies and deep appreciation for anyone who didn't make the final cut.

Lastly, sincere thanks to Alice and Oliver at Aeon Books for committing to this text—and waiting for it!

PREFACE

There have been many excellent commentaries on plant medicine, herbal medicine, herbalism, phytotherapy, to mention some of the names under which such discussions present themselves. Why do we need another one? What does this book hope to offer in addition to the ones that we already have?

It may be easier to describe what this book is not, before attempting to describe what it is—or aspires to be. It is not a *materia medica*, a collection of monographs of plants in common medicinal use. It is not a historical or cultural account of Herbal Medicine. It is not an instruction manual for a particular specific herbal medicine school or tradition. It is not a theoretical medicinal tract listing clinical applications driven by an accepted epistemology of clinical sciences. It is not a practical manual on how to "do" herbal medicine—although many practical tips may be included. Lastly, it is not a book about Plant Spirit Medicine (though it may come close), no matter that that study and practice has been constitutional in deepening my own relationship to plants, to Nature, and to the business of writing about these things.

Although I enter the discussion from a specific perspective—that of a herbalist (I use plants, professionally, in a healing practice)—I am not in this volume promoting that practice. In fact, to some extent I will be interrogating it. You will read, in Chapter 3, about the epiphany that brought me to professional herbal medicine practice. I strongly suspect that plants were not merely the object of that epiphany but had agency in promoting it. If that is true, why did they do so? Because they cared enough about me to hand me my career on a plate? Or for some hitherto unrevealed motive of their own? And if the latter, what might that look like? There is a significant challenge here to the perspective and the narrative of human-centredness. I will have much to say about this, and about the agency of plants throughout this book.

This is a book about the deep, enduring, and *necessary* relationship between humans and plants. It is a book about the heart-centredness of a natural association that is driven by a definable world-view—a philosophy if you like, although without the unnecessary complexity of thought that that term implies. It seeks to inculcate, to honour, and to develop within its readers a feeling of deep gratitude and love towards the system of reality that has thrown us together in cohabitation, collaboration, and symbiosis. And it seeks to place the various actors, or agents, in that symbiosis, on equal footing with each other.

Nature is not what most people think of it—something "out there", apart from us, but which we can "visit" occasionally to make us feel better. Nor is it simply something green, something wild, something dangerous, something scary. It is all those things, but it is far more. Nature is always ever-present *within us*. It *is* us, as surely as it is the plants, the Earth, and all her creatures. We are constantly cradled, nourished, connected, animated, and vitalised by Nature, whether we recognise it or not. Nature is the reason we are alive. And this world, the entire collaborative construct, the planet and all its denizens, plant, animal, insect, fungi—the clades and phyla of biological classification, together with the environment that supports them—is the living evidence of the virtually limitless creativity of Nature.

The medicine of plants is proposed as an answer—or part of an answer—to the problem, or the *perception*, of human alienation in modernity. Alienation from the natural world and from the other species with which we cohabit. Alienation, ultimately, from *ourselves*, our true nature—whatever that is—and certainly from each other. Plants, perhaps along with animals, may represent a point of entry for the human into the realm of the non-human. They are both conducive and convivial. We have a relationship of convenience with them. They perform special functions for us, and thus we are able to recognise them and have an ontologically stable relationship with them. Similarly, animals. Different animals, different plants, different purposes. Animals and plants who share our space—home and garden. We might talk to them, even regard them as quasi-human. Animals and plants that we consume. Animals and plants that we revile and eschew. What is the difference?

The hierarchy that we habitually ascribe to that system is a construct, generated by an ontology—or world-view—that is specific to our current cultural orientation, but which is not necessarily natively human. What if we were able to conceptualise a structure in which there is no hierarchy? What if we are being challenged to drop our conceit and give up being the King of the Castle in this shared domain? How many of us know what that might even mean?

Shaun Ellis, "The Man Who Lives with Wolves", spent two years in the wild as a member of a wolf pack.[1] He didn't do it by wading into the midst of their circle and "subduing" them with his superior human intelligence. He subjugated himself. He was not too proud to become the lowliest member of the pack—the one everyone else had a go at when they in turn were being chastised by their governing individuals. He learned the language of submission. It was necessary for his survival in that setting. Human arrogance would have seen him finished off in a matter of hours. The Nez Perce Indians of Idaho who had given him directions thought he was a lunatic and predicted that he would never come back. Eighteen months later he returned to their settlement, ready to teach the world what he had learned from the wolves.

Contemporaneously, consumption is predicated upon commodification. We are going to have to confront that as part of this enquiry. Humans have carefully constructed a world in which we are ourselves largely immune from the danger of being consumed—in the obvious sense, at least. But we are, in fact, consummate consumers of everything, including ourselves. We are slaves to a system (capitalism) that places everything in subordination to the endgame of making money (for the few, not for the many), and on whose account we use ourselves up daily, delivering unending service in a continuing act of self-immolation. We have commodified ourselves, our worth measured in economic valency and means-tested to destruction. The unthinking and concupiscent consumption of the natural world and its resources—which is a symptom of our deepest sickness, the objectification of the world and of ourselves—is by necessity also the underlying factor in our lack of regard for *Soul*, not in the sense of a religious commodity that we might "lose" if we do not behave as priests dictate, but in the sense of our vital connection with *All That Is*. The source of everything and the vital energy within.

There is such a thing as "plant blindness", or *Plant Awareness Disparity*—the tendency among humans to ignore, under-appreciate, or remain unaware, of the existence of plants. Despite the fact that most of us eat plants daily, sit on furniture made out of plants, wear fabric made out of plants, use them to decorate our gardens and our homes, probably curse them when they grow where they "shouldn't", and most importantly perhaps breathe oxygen that has been largely manufactured by them, the average person among us has little interest in their reality, their diversity, their particular kind of consciousness, or their critical role in maintaining life on our planet.

The consequences of plant blindness are far-reaching: limited interest in and funding for plant conservation, the dwindling numbers of educational programmes in plant sciences, leading to the failure to protect our plant co-habitants from industrial exploitation, poisoning, genetic modification, criminal activity and the insidious land-grabbing of a money-hungry economic regime. Dr Carly Cowell, writing for the website of the Royal Botanical Gardens at Kew, offers scientific explanations for this phenomenon, citing theory that suggests that as hunter gatherers we learned to prioritise colours other than green in our fight to stay ahead of animal predators, but also talks about the "nature deficit disorder which is the alienation of people from the natural environment".[2]

Whatever the causes are, I hope through the pages of this book to convince the reader that addressing this imbalance is a survival issue, for the individual and for the species. Scenarios of fully artificial civilisations, while making for exciting science fiction, rarely (even in fiction) translate to enhanced quality of life, physical and psychological health, or the self-determination of individuals or populations. Our world, at this critical juncture in human history, is one in which assets that should belong to all are controlled by vested interests, and wealth is syphoned in a continuing stream to the apex of the fiscal pyramid. It is one in which we are fed and medicated by the artificial products that sustain the wealth and the power base of self-selecting elite members of our race. And it is one in which plants, animals and humans are sacrificed to the insatiable greed and emptiness of a system that no longer has a spiritual heart. This world is no longer a fiction: it is imminently upon us and embedding itself slowly deeper, day by day—unless we have the courage to stop, to pluck out the rot and change direction.

The word *medicine*, also, needs expansion. Is it just stuff you put down your throat in the expectation of cure, or even simply the relief of symptoms? Is it nothing more than blister packs and brands, than the technologised interventions of the surgeon? Even than witches' potions and unguents? Is it more than the World Health Organization definition of health, widely thought to give that institution a credibility that is arguably suspect in light of recent global events?[3] Can we inscribe medicine into our intention as a catalyst to the deep experience of wholeness that we all crave, and which we all seek, albeit sometimes in perverse, terrifying and destructive ways? Is not Medicine that which opens our hearts, elevates us and restores our connection with *soul*? In the story that I hope will unfold through these pages, I will argue that plants are well placed to do precisely this by virtue of also being ensouled.

It's a big ask. What has the attrition of human activity on the planet to do with the other denizens with whom we share the space? Why should they help us? And what might we owe them for their trouble? Most challenging of all, if all enjoined beings co-curate this physical space, what is *their* role in producing the effects that we complain of? It is often said, we need Nature; Nature does not need us. But is that true? Is Nature not suffering because part of it—the human—has become sick? And if allopathic intervention is considered suppressive, then the mere removal of the human is not going to effect the cure, any more than the removal of the tumour would guarantee that it will not return, and with double or treble the destructive force of the original lesion.

The same reasoning might be pressed into service in consideration of one of my own *bête noires*: the presence among us, referred to extensively in Chapter 1, of a parasitic class of human agents whose subtle, almost unnoticed rise to absolute influence, wealth and power now lies behind almost every major geopolitical issue that we face. Corporate industrialists and self-made oligarchs, framed as "philanthropists" by many, but denied their very humanity by others,[4] men (usually) who, once we have seen through the ruse of philanthropy, can either be vilified and scapegoated, or rehabilitated as those who arrived here to teach us a lesson—no matter that in doing so they have also enmired themselves in deep opprobrium and censure. It's not looking good for them, on the level of simple human ethics and morality, and it's not going to get any better. That's some sacrifice. They have chosen to embody the shadow side of humanity: the avarice, the cold, calculating self-interest, the unassuageable hunger for power, and the predilection towards cruelty and abuse.

According to the *Law of One*,[5] there is Service to Others, and there is Service to Self. The major religions of the world usually have in common that service to others is the Golden Rule. Service to Self (the domain of Satan, or Lucifer, perhaps) is a lesser regarded path, but many see it as a viable one—at least up to a point. Ultimately there is no "self" and "other", and therefore service is simply service, even though conducted in a manner that appears superficially loathsome and reprehensible. Every story needs a villain, right?

The lesson is to withdraw our support for what we do not prefer—and thereby reclaim our power. But we must also understand it, for there, but for the grace of *All That Is*, we may also go, until, perhaps, we learn the meaning of *enlightened self-interest*—whereby the difference between self and other is effaced by the notion that my best interest is also your best interest, and that of the community as a whole—and by that I mean the entire global community of terrestrial species, as perhaps also the galactic community of beings we have not yet even encountered, but to whom, some say, we may need to answer in the fulness of time.

In the plant world "allelopathic (chemical) warfare" is a recognised phenomenon. This is where a plant may deliberately and systematically kill nearby members of its own or other species, through the release of toxic chemicals into the root systems. But allelopathy is usually recognised as a biologically coherent survival mechanism in cases where for example the proliferation of individuals threatens survival of the species in the immediate environment. It has been shown, to take one example, that the root exudates of Manchurian walnut (*Juglans mandshurica*) significantly reduce the growth rate of its own seedlings. So much so that plantations of the species fare better when other plants, such as larch, are introduced alongside them, in contrast to homogenous plantations.[6]

A commentary on this, however, brings out another key thread in the thesis of this book. Plantations are a human construction, and an endeavour generally embarked upon in the pursuit of commercial aims. Are we seeing in this phenomenon the botanical equivalent of "political" resistance to a colonialist threat, enshrined in an endemic and resident biochemical capability? And if so, what does this say about our own political aspirations, including those that may lead to warfare and the subjugation of others?

Dan Quinn's eponymous gorilla protagonist, Ishmael, says something quite similar: he points out that territorialism among tribes is a biological necessity. Tolerance towards migrants is an existential threat in a situation where availability of space and food is the algorithmic function of survival.[7] Such principles are of course widely observed in animal behaviour, but we tend to think of ourselves as "above" that kind of behaviour. Even while deprecating the arrival of immigrants onto our own shores.

The problem with such declarations of expediency, however, is that they have been, and are being used to justify some of the worst kinds of human behaviour: racism, apartheid, eugenics, genocide. The concept of the "useless eater" arose in Nazi Germany as a description of disabled people, and was invoked as justification for exterminating 240,000 of them in the same camps that also oversaw the demise of six million Jews.[8] But the term also appears as a chapter heading in Linda André's *Doctors of Deception.*[9] André charts the advance of psychiatry in the USA, specifically in the context of the application of ECT as a corrective therapy, and notes complicity on the part of highly respected industrialists of the late 19th and early 20th centuries—Kellogg, Eastman, Rockefeller, Carnegie—in campaigns of eugenics directed towards people with mental health problems. The influence—and the descendants—of these giants of industry, it should be remembered, are still alive and well in the current era, and are found infiltrating some of our most prominent institutions of global governance, including the World Economic Forum and the World Health Organization. Watch closely debates on population control, and you may have cause to reflect that some of our fellow human beings appear to have very definite ideas about who is or is not worthy to live alongside them on this planet.

But within one plant species, is there a case of a single individual, or an oligarchy of individuals, demanding obeisance on pain of deprivation or extermination on a widespread scale? Imagine a huge dandelion suddenly arising out of the mass of little dandelions. Maybe he has discovered a new way to transport nutrients along root systems and is now controlling the available supply of necessary goods, taking far more than his fair share. The other dandelions first worship him as a god, a saviour, even, and then realise that he is slowly starving them, and depriving them of their basic self-determination. How do they rebel? How do they secure their safety and independence from the monster?

An anthropomorphic morality tale, for sure, and one of highly unlikely proportions. One of the cautions, when approaching an understanding of plants, as of any other non-human species, is that we may err in projecting human traits and human emotions onto these entities. I find this to be the case frequently in the practice of what is known as 'Plant Spirit Medicine', where one manifestation of this is in the assigning of gender to plants. I have listened to endless impassioned arguments among students as to whether such and such a plant spirit is male or female. I generally sigh and remind them, only a little disingenuously, that plant sexuality is botanically complicated, and that any other assignation of gender is at best fanciful and hugely subjective. We will return to this at a later stage, when discussing our personal relationships with plants, and although it is possible that the choice of visualisation has a lot more to do with us than it does the plant, the gendering of plants is a phenomenon that is deeply embedded in contexts where the role of plants in human society is fully recognised and honoured, such as the indigenous communities of the Amazon rainforest. It is worthy of some deeper investigation, and we will consider the implications later in this book.

But perhaps the best way to reinvent our connection with plants is via the age-old method of storytelling. Plants occupied a special position in pre-technological societies, and we don't have to go back too far to see this in action. From the Nine Herbs Charm of the Anglo Saxons to the poetry of Shakespeare, we find the cultural currency of plants rife and redolent in the literature and the folklore of our land, with many resonances and symbolisms now long forgotten. Were such ideas inherent in, indeed *generated* by the nature of the plants themselves? Or were they fanciful, and ephemeral, human projections? And more than that, why do we not, in our own age, have similarly rich symbolic representations when it comes to plants?

There's rosemary, that's for remembrance;
Pray you, love, remember.
And there is pansies; that's for thoughts.
There's fennel for you, and columbines.
There's rue for you; and here's some
for me: we may call it herb of grace a' Sundays.

You may wear your rue with a difference.
There's a daisy. I would give you some violets,
but they withered all when my father died.
They say he made a good end.[10]

This from Shakespeare's *Hamlet*. Ophelia in her "madness"—a psychological and emotional crisis triggered by the death of her father, Polonius, but also by her painful awareness of the seeming impossibility of bringing the murderers to justice. "Something is rotten in the state of Denmark", mutters the palace guard, after the ghost of the dead king, Hamlet's father, appears on the parapet. In the famous painting by John Everett Millais, Ophelia drowns almost serenely, bestrewn with her plant allies and clutching a posy in her right hand. How would plants in our era inform the stories that would reveal the true state of things here? Perhaps this is what I am reaching for in writing this book also as a personal story of my own involvement, and my attempt, over years and decades, to make that involvement as consciously aware, and as *ethical*, as possible.

There are many stories as we move through the chapters of this book. Some of them are personal. Many of them come from the interweaving of human histories with those of plants. Chapter 2 deals with the matter of what we might owe our plant companions on earth, and how we might redeem those debts. Chapters 3 addresses the nature of Nature itself, and Chapters 4, 5 and 6 discuss the various parameters of what we call "medicine". These chapters open up a metaphysical debate that I see as a necessary counterpart and antidote to modernity as an ontological, as well as a historiographic concept, and invite us to see beyond what we are taught to believe, the received and endlessly reiterated narratives of an age where control and profit are the chief institutional—and constitutional—forces.

Chapter 7 delves into the possibility of communicating with the entities that we know as plants, and proposes a template for understanding this possibility by reference to the metaphysics already alluded to, while in Chapter 8 we get to meet the Master Plants themselves, those beings who have made it their own unique trajectory to interact with humans in era-defining ways. Chapter 9 is devoted to the practicalities of communicating with plants, giving tried and tested methods of managing those interactions; and finally, Chapter 10 invites us to step up to planetary citizenship and consider how we may offer our own unique medicine for the benefit of all beings with whom we share this realm.

I warn my readers of two things here. One, that I have woven elements of my own story into the fabric of the book, chapter on chapter. I see this as nailing my colours to the mast, and I hope it adds colour and context, drawn as it is from the life of someone who has devoted more than 40 years to healing with plants. Secondly, that I choose to begin, in Chapter 1, with a brief account of some of what I see to be problematic in the current state of affairs that we must contend with. If we are to allow ourselves to be rescued by the agency of plants, it is as well that we know what from, and how plants can be, as I believe they seek to be, the intuitive heroes of the moment. By the end of the book I hope I can provide a framework for thinking this through, and offer my own pantheon of botanical heroes, with whom I and others work regularly in healing ourselves and others, and by extension, the planet itself.

The healing, however, is always *within* us—it IS us, just as much as it is "nature", for we ARE nature. We are merely ushered into its presence by those beings that have not forgotten that fact. Plants, ancient co-evolvers and co-creators in the physical system of reality that we inhabit, are the ones who have not forgotten.

Notes

1. Ellis, S. & Junor, P. (2010). *The Man Who Lives with Wolves.* New York: Three Rivers Press.
2. Cowell, C. (2020). Plant Blindness and Conservation Implications. Retrieved from: https://www.kew.org/read-and-watch/plant-blindness-conservation-implications.
3. "Health is a state of complete physical, mental and social well-being and not merely the absence of disease or infirmity." https://www.who.int/about/governance/constitution.
4. Narratives that cast such individuals as 'reptilian' or 'extraterrestrial' abound in the marginal literature of our time, evidencing an all-too-common human proclivity to project our shadow onto a carefully circumscribed "other".
5. Elkins, D., Rueckert, C., McCarty, J. (2018). *The Ra Contact: Teaching the Law of One*, Volumes 1 & 2. Louisville KY: L/L Research.
6. Yang, L., Wang, P., Kong C. H. (2010). Effect of Larch (*Larix gmelini* Rupr.) Root Exudates on Manchurian Walnut (*Juglans mandshurica* Maxim.) Growth and Soil Juglone in a Mixed-species Plantation. *Plant and Soil, 329*(1): 249–258.

7. Quinn, D. (2009). *Ishmael*. New York: Bantam.
8. Mostert, M. (2002). Useless Eaters: Disability as Genocidal Marker in Nazi Germany. *The Journal of Special Education, 36*(3): 155–168.
9. André, L. (2019). *Doctors of Deception*. New Brunswick: Rutgers University Press.
10. Shakespeare's *Hamlet*, Act IV, Scene 5.

CHAPTER ONE

Of carbon and frogs: escaping the cauldron

> *Someday you will die, and somehow something's gonna steal your carbon.*
>
> Modest Mouse[1]

I was five years old when I first stayed at *Elfins*, and twelve years old by the time that experience came to an end with the untimely death of my grandfather. The cottage sat in a slight hollow, wrapped around to the rear by a bank of tall trees and stretching down to The Common, a minor thoroughfare that ran through the Sussex village of West Chiltington on its way to the nearby town of Pulborough. The garden was long, so long that, entering it from the road onto a gravel standing for vehicles, the cottage itself could not be seen until you had ventured about 50 yards up the path that ran up one side, past the large thuja which stood sentry approximately in the centre of the grounds, to where the sweeping lawns descended in terraces, and the front elevation finally came into view, along (in season) with a vibrant display of summer flowers—my grandfather especially prized delphiniums and lupins.

The top lawn was an immaculate rectangle that was frequently commissioned for the playing of croquet—a genteel summer pastime that belied our relatively humble social status—and was bordered on all sides with beds featuring aubretia, alyssum, marigold and lavender, with spikes of the taller plants, alliums and gladioli alongside the beloved lupins and delphiniums.

The lower lawn was less formal, sloping to a thick border boasting a majestic holly tree, alongside quince, azalia and japonica, which curved around, leaving the great conifer to the right, to reveal a third lower lawn with a well-stocked fishpond (goldfish and frogspawn) encircled by a rockery occupied by thyme, sempervivum, campanula and saxifrage.

Further down from this, going back towards the gravel vehicle standing, the small garage and the entrance gate, four rows of sweet peas and garden vegetables—runner and dwarf beans, tomatoes, courgettes and marrows—provided a good portion of the food that we enjoyed at my grandmother's table during our stay, but that was not the total vegetable count. Back up around the house, light gravel pathways circled the cottage—the greater portion of which dated back to the 18th century, featuring cast iron Suffolk latches and tongue and groove doors—and led to the rear garden, cradled by a bank of rhododendron and tall trees—ash, I think—at the border. Here was the vegetable garden proper: onions, carrots, potatoes, a variety of brassicas—brussels sprouts, cabbage, broccoli, cauliflower—and, hard up against the rear wall of the cottage, a glass cucumber frame, which I seem to remember being the source of several cautionary injunctions during child-filled visits—during the years that I knew the place there were eventually five of us, myself and my siblings, as well as cousins, nieces and nephews of various denominations, regularly visiting.

In the rear garden were two structures that held great fascination for us as children. One was the presence of a "witch's house" at the rear border, under its canopy of ivy and overhanging branches. This was a moss-encrusted stone arch leading to a shallow but dark, dank cave-like space that we rarely dared enter. Apparently, a local historical fact sheet referred to two of these, but I remember only one. It sent frissons of fear and excitement in equal measure through our naïve young sensibilities, and, once warned of its purpose and nature, was something we hardly ever mentioned or talked about.

The other was my grandfather's "shed". It was actually more of a barn, a great, overlapped, creosoted galleon of a building that was distinctly Tardis-like on the inside. It was full of subdivisions of rooms, each with a different focus and purpose, from garden tools and storage to woodworking and DIY, to man-cave private space. I was certainly privileged to enter this hallowed space, and even more so when my grandfather showed me, or occasionally shared with me, magic tricks. He was a member of the Magic Circle, and an accomplished magician—although we would more accurately call him a conjurer—and he possessed the full paraphernalia, comprising playing cards (both straight and prepared), silk handkerchiefs, wands, top hats, watches, coins, crystal balls, and a magnificent black cloak, fastened with a dazzling golden clasp below the chin. The only missing items were the white rabbit and the doves.

But the real magic of my grandfather was his green fingers. He could seemingly make anything grow, and the sheer wealth of plant life in this altogether magical domain was awe-inspiring indeed to my young self. When he died, unexpectedly, of a heart attack (in his GP's office—nice touch, Grandpa), I was desolate. It was the end of an era.

* * *

We are at a point in the history of the human where a clear choice is beginning to emerge. Perhaps this has been going on for some time—it does not matter how long, although the historians may one day argue about it—that is, if there is anyone left to argue about it. For many this choice is enshrined in the urgency of impending climate catastrophe and what needs to be done to avert it. For others this is a superficial gloss on a far deeper problem.

By appearing to call climate change 'superficial' I do not mean to dismiss or relegate its importance. But confusion abounds, not only about the real meaning of "net zero", but upon the aetiology of the problem itself, and certainly when it comes to the plethora of fixes being put forward. Hypocrisy, hidden agendas and double-speak are rife among law- and policy-makers, such that it seems once again that, as in wars, recessions and pandemics, the consequences devolve primarily onto those already under pressure of poverty, illness and political disenfranchisement, not to say gaslighting and scapegoating.

In 1959, Winfried Otto Schumann mathematically predicted the discovery of electromagnetic frequencies generated by the earth itself. The Schumann Resonances range from 3Hz to 60Hz, and peak at definable intervals in response to natural excitatory events such as lightning strikes, seismic activity, and solar perturbations of the ionosphere. They arise owing to the closed system operating between the earth's surface and the ionosphere, which forms a resonant cavity for extremely low-frequency electromagnetic wavelengths. The lowest frequency—3Hz—is the wavelength of the circumference of the planet itself and forms the background of all frequencies experienced on our world, but regular spikes at 7.38Hz are noted and have been dubbed the "heartbeat of the planet". There is some evidence to suggest that this frequency is salutary for all life forms on the planet and is, for humans, "linked to improved cognitive functions, reduced stress and anxiety, enhanced immune function, sleep function, and much more".[2]

In terms of human impacts on these resonant fields, it is known that the experiments in atmospheric excitation conducted at the HAARP (High-frequency Active Auroral Research Program) facility in Alaska can impact the Schumann resonances.[3] Among other as yet unverified (or unadmitted) anthropogenic impacts are the use of thermobaric weapons, and the discovery of "exotic particles" in the LHC (Large Hadron Collider) facility at Cern.[4] I have offered the opinion elsewhere that if we want to be exhaustive in our analysis of the phenomenon of human-driven climate change, then carbon emissions must take their place among other potential candidates. Punching holes in the ionosphere, deliberately or inadvertently "modifying" weather patterns, and messing with the building blocks of physical reality itself, while simultaneously settling on just one officially endorsed culprit, is at best disingenuous, at worst criminally negligent or culpable.

But can we go further? Can we hypothesise that humans may be causal in spiking the resonant frequencies of the earth, not only via technology, but by means of changes or fluctuations in their own resonant frequencies? All beings have their electromagnetic frequencies, and within those beings, specific organs also resonate at their own frequencies, in complex, constantly interacting patterns of harmony or interference.[5] The health or otherwise of an organ is not merely a local event. Everything affects everything else, all the time. Might not the convulsions that we see taking place at any point in history, natural disasters, war and famine, feed macroscopically into this soup of electromagnetic affects?

> *The universe is the aggregate of all of humanity's consciously-apprehended and communicated experience with the non-simultaneous, nonidentical, and only partially overlapping, always complementary, weigh-able and unweigh-able, ever omni-transforming, event sequences* (R. Buckminster Fuller).[6]

What if one answer to global warming is a reduction in *human* warming? What if the frogs in the cauldron[7] are not being boiled simply by a preponderance of carbon in the composition of the atmosphere, but also by other factors hitherto undiagnosed? What if they—we—are being overheated and driven insane by our own cultural milieu? It is this field of harmonic chaos, the electromagnetic signature of human distress, confusion and insanity, generated by core psychological dissonances maintained by regimes of fear, impotence, impoverishment and oppression, which the natural world also registers and to which it attempts, as it must, to entrain itself. Perhaps symptom and cause in climate change is a faulty collective psychological gestalt, self-proliferating in an escalating positive feedback spiral. Perhaps the perceived contribution of technologically induced incoherence is a symptom of far deeper currents of actualisation, arising within the human soul itself, and requiring a commensurate adaptation within the energy fields of cohabiting entities of all denominations, up to and including the earth itself? Physical overheating as an analogue of psychological overheating?

There is a familiar expectation that problems created by human technology will also be solved by human technology. The industrialists liked it when we bought cars, holidays, gadgets, pills—when we *consumed*. They got us hooked on it all, and let's face it, it made them rich. Unconscionably rich. Then the problems attendant upon these things began to become evident, and we now must take on board that consumption is, after all, bad—or rather that the old things we consumed are no longer approved of; that we must now break those addictions and instead get addicted to new stuff. Less problematic stuff—supposedly. But still stuff by which industrialists continue to get rich. *Plus ça change.*

"Problems cannot be solved with the same mindset that created them."[8] The new "solutions" almost invariably issue from the same mindset as the old problems. The truth is that the mindset and the science are one, woven from the same cloth. Solutions to climate change almost exclusively rest upon the imperative to "cut the carbon" at all costs. Zero emissions, the economy of suppression, a band aid plastered over a long-standing chronic illness.

And yet even while promulgating the case that human-generated carbon emissions are at cause in accelerating the predicted climate catastrophe, scratch the surface on nation state rationales for skirmishes, conflicts and wars over the last half a century since climate warnings began to enter public and policy debate, and you will find that control of the global fossil fuel market is almost invariably lurking there among other nefarious motives. The Gulf War, Iraq, Libya, Sudan, Russia–Ukraine, the US sanctions, and as I write, bombing campaigns and impending "regime change" in Venezuela in defence of the petrodollar;[9] and not least, the rich deposits of oil and gas off the coast of Gaza, upon which Israel and the West have set their entitled, imperialist sights, along with the current fracas focussed on the Strait of Hormuz in the Persian Gulf. Whatever other rationales are deployed to justify the use of unconscionable military force and the wholesale shedding of blood, control of global energy supplies is usually in evidence, even if only as an incidental benefit of conquest. More than this, military operations themselves account for 5.5% of global emissions—a share larger than civilian air travel and maritime transport combined.[10] We will see other examples of rampant and ballooning energy use in a few moments.

To be clear (and possibly unpopular), simply reducing carbon will never be successful while the old mindset prevails. Unless the carbon they want to reduce is … us? We all breathe out carbon dioxide. We ARE carbon, animated carbon. *Someday you will die, and somehow something's gonna steal your carbon*. They're on it already, they haven't even waited for us to die—or rather, they are doing what they can to hasten the day. Paranoid? Maybe. But a quick look around this place will, as I have discussed elsewhere,[11] reveal a thousand and one potential sources of death lurking in everyday utilities such as water, food and medicines, household products, agrochemicals and industrial effluent, and in the very air that we breathe. These are not accidental side effects of modern life: they are deliberately placed in our environment by people who are profiting insanely from their continued use, even after the ill-effects have been widely recognised and commented on. Even while lawsuits have been fought and won on the back of such claims.[12]

Meanwhile these same self-entitled fellow humans of ours continue to run their private jets, limousines, diesel super-yachts and multiple mansions. I could not aspire to a carbon footprint like theirs in a thousand lifetimes such as the one I inhabit. This is not envy: it is incredulity—and, I admit it, disgust. Not at the practice itself, but at the hypocrisy and entitlement of the assumptions that lie at the base of it: "One rule for us, another for you. We deserve these things, you do not. You must take climate change seriously, we don't have to."

The "new stuff" that we are enjoined to buy, the techno-solutions, are all too often still problematic, even in the same terms that the old stuff was. Take the internet—the unavoidable facilitator of reduced transportation needs, among other major lifestyle adjustments (not to say curtailments) we are being asked to make. Everyone is busy logging on to it, uploading to it, backing up to it, uploading their lives to it, ordering goods and take-away food with it, not to mention validating and calibrating themselves by reference to its resident approved pantheon of administrators, adjudicators, influencers, and fact-checkers—many of these no longer even human. Increasingly, we are utterly dependent on it. Information technology has been quietly assuming numerous functions that previously required physical relocation using transportation systems. Ordering groceries, going to the bank to cash cheques, even going to work. We found that out in the pandemic. I was never busier, creating remote content for my classes, seeing my patients online when I could not see them face to face. I was grateful enough for the tech at that era. I still am. I think.

So, what of it? The Cloud seems such an effortless resource, such an elegant solution to the problem of data storage. The reality is somewhat different. Clouds of this denomination do not float prettily in the sky. They take up huge amounts of very physical space—even though sometimes in the middle of deserts—and (here's the elephant) HUMONGOUS amounts of ENERGY. They are among the most impactful activities in environmental terms, with an overall carbon footprint bigger than that of the airline industry.[13] A single data centre is estimated to consume the equivalent of the power needed to supply 50,000 ordinary homes. In 2019 70% of the world's internet traffic used facilities in Virginia's "data center alley", facilities that are, it turns out, heavily reliant on "dirty" (carbon-based) energy supplies.

And it's not just the power to run the computing operations: 40% of the power used for these plants is needed for cooling. The more data is processed, the more heat is generated, and the more cooling is necessary. The cooling process also uses hundreds of millions of gallons of water—something else they are already warning will be in short supply in our comfortable "developed" world very soon. It has been estimated that, for each kilowatt hour of energy a data centre consumes, two litres of water are needed for cooling. Will we be thirsty because machines need to drink?

Now add to that the exponential development of artificial intelligence—"generative AI" as we call it now. Between 2022 and 2023 the power requirements of data centres in North America increased by a hundred percent.[14] Most of the increase was accounted for by the phenomenal rise of advanced computing solutions known collectively as AI, and since AI appears to be progressing in the direction of limitless growth, it is logical to expect that energy and water consumption will follow the same pattern.

I am acutely conscious as I write that, as a Cloud user, and as someone who has recently, despite deep reservations, dipped into using AI for specific, targeted tasks, this text will itself be adding, if microscopically, to that load—the ever-increasing allostatic load bearing on the homeostatic mechanisms of earth's ecosystem. The irony is not lost on me, but in this case, irony is more than a figure of speech. It is increasingly a trap from which it is difficult to escape. It seems to my wholly inexpert opinion that we are being driven from one eco-wrecking set of habits and expectations to another potentially far worse one. Whatever happened to pen and paper? Could I even perform the act of writing a book that way anymore? And how much of a Luddite am I prepared to be? And that's before we go anywhere near the question of what, in fact, AI is, and what it may be doing to our very humanity.

The World Wide Web, and its supporting hardware, is a matrix that is slowly and surely enveloping (enslaving?) us all—has been for a couple of decades now. And although on the one hand ever larger numbers of people have been able to access enhanced opportunities for education, information and personal empowerment, it has simultaneously enabled greater levels of influence, indoctrination, financial and political control, and globalist and trans-humanist agendas. Novels have been written about it—and not just recently. From Samuel Butler's *Erewhon* (1872), through the infamous Borg of Gene Roddenberry's *Star Trek* (1966 through the latter 20th century) to Dan Brown's *Origin* (2017) and *The Secret of Secrets* (2025), the human imagination has prefigured days when either man and machine become merged, or machines themselves develop consciousness. Some might say they have invoked this—imagination is, after all, generative.[15] As Yuval Noah Harari observes, the power to divide the human world into the two polar constituencies, the technologically enhanced "superelite" and the unreconstructed and therefore obsolete "useless masses", is in the hands of those who control the algorithms.[16] Harari's contention is that *Homo sapiens sapientis* (the wisest of the wise) is not long for this world. To be replaced by?

This tension between that which our strident and cacophonous world tells us we are, and the song that, try as we might to block it out and avert our ears, many of us still hear insistently from the depths of our authentic being, especially when among natural phenomena—gardens, meadows, forests, hills, rivers, lakes, oceans, mountains and deep expanses of azure sky—is constitutional to the contemporary sensibility. The modern way, the grid of culture, mandate and prohibition, aided and abetted by technology, coexists peculiarly and uneasily with the ancient way, which is rooted in the ever flowing and changing rhythms of the unfolding, immanent nature of life and soul.

The Druids had a name for it: *Awen*, the "flowing spirit".[17] It is too easy—and dangerous—to claim that this no longer operates, that we have finally all but succeeded in eradicating the organic immanence of life in favour of something more predictable, more governable, more *controllable*. We can see all too clearly, despite our ingenuity, that Nature still has ways of defeating our best-laid plans. Does Awen flow through machines? It is a question whose answer is perhaps not as predictable as you may think. In the end, however, I would rather be one of Harari's useless masses than a member of his superelite. By the end of this book, I hope you will understand why, if you don't already.

Wyrd, often described as fate, or consequence, is a concept from the old Norse spirituality, which speaks of an interconnecting force that binds all phenomena such that the slightest action on any one part instantly affects the whole. I guess it's similar to the Indic philosophical notion of Karma. We forget that there was once a towering metaphysics in these Northern lands. To transgress the laws of Wyrd is to invite unwanted consequences. Wyrd is the force that eventually destroys the lives of the violators of "unknowable" universal order.[18] On the other hand, to live in the flow of Wyrd is to enable the hero's journey and quest, the victorious attainment of the desired outcome.

In modern-day parlance we might invoke, as an explanatory mechanism, the interweaving electromagnetic fields generated by all bodies—biologically "alive" or not, from molecules, microbes and single cells, plants, animals and humans, to rocks, rivers, oceans, hills, planets, stars, galaxies and supermassive black holes—and the varying levels of coherence between those fields that may move individuals towards conflict and dissonance, or towards convergence and harmony.

Or we might invoke the diaphanous quantum concepts of non-locality and entanglement. Ultimately unity—and harmony—is assured. It cannot be otherwise within the ONE. That is also the ultimate nature of Wyrd. However, down here in the maelstrom we'd better hope that someone who knows their shit has got the helm: these are choppy waters indeed at this earthbound, quarter-century locus in time and space.

Humans have been absolute in asserting our pre-eminence in the world. "Recorded" history is precisely the attempt to solidify our achievements and recursively reinforce the foundations, the template and the justification, for the world that we have built and, some might say, in which we have trapped ourselves, along (maybe) with the other living species with whom we share it. And although it has been millennia in the making, this world has latterly received a turbo-boost on the back of technological advancements that are unprecedented within our current cultural reach and its historiographic anamnesis. It is important, in the maintaining of cognitive coherence, to ensure that we get the originary story straight; and indeed, the success of this editing and reclassifying of the past is clearly evident in the fact that hardly anyone questions it.

We might observe that there are two matrices operating at this time. Awen and Wyrd have a competitor. The Matrix is more than the obvious technological frameworks that give rise to the Internet of Things. It is far older. It is the legislative, fiscal and educational structures, the geopolitical grids that divide physical space on the planet, and the medical structures—the kind of medicine that arose, as Foucault observed, when writing became involved, and men of science began "botanizing in the field of pathology".[19] The contemporary Matrix is a construct that *appears* to be independent of construction. It is imbricated into the psychological structure of the populace such that they do not notice it: it's just the way things are.

We can see this playing out in so many ways, if we look hard enough. Few people question the fact that their identity is inscribed in the processes of legislative and governmental machinery, and that it is this fact, uniquely, that enables taxation, accountability to authority, eligibility to education, social security and medical attention, and access to vital services such as water, power, communication, transport, money, and even food. The "straw man" is a version of you created, purportedly, to make your life easier, to protect and shield you from adversity, to ensure you have whatever you need in life; but in reality also to ensure compliance with social and legal norms, and to legitimise the seizing of your assets, either by the stealth of taxation, by legal injunction, or (coming soon) by means of the power invested in the Central Bank Digital Currency to cancel your entitlement to money altogether, should you transgress. Digital ID is its harbinger. Digitise individuals so that effectively they no longer exist as emancipated beings, but instead are part of the very fabric of an orchestrated technological prison. They won't even have to police us anymore: we are already policed by ourselves and each other, and increasingly by an impersonal system that is seemingly answerable to no one, and with an alarming decrease in the right of appeal.

The deeper question of who you in fact ARE, in your greater metaphysical reality, is not something you are encouraged to be concerned with. And if you do find yourself pondering and searching, it can always be sold back to you by means of a self-generating and self-replicating industry of self-discovery and self-improvement methods, which stand in contemporary relation to the masses in the way that religion once did. Again, prescriptive, coercive, prohibitive, punitive and reclamatory—a continual looping back into temporal power and institutional control, done in ways that neatly sidestep our attempts to penetrate the veil, while offering a simulation of sublimity that we are increasingly unable to distinguish from the real thing—whatever that is. And always the paywall. *Ker-ching!*

The Matrix—the film version—is a latter-day allegory for the quest for liberation and individuation, in the Jungian sense. The hero's journey and triumph, his mastery over hitherto unseen forces that hold the masses in thrall; the jettisoning of the veil of unknowing and of the restrictive enchantment of the artificial world of appearances; the coming of age into full human capability and the attainment of invincibility. The hero, Neo, having been sprung from the Matrix by Morpheus and his resistance, undergoes rigorous training in martial arts as part of his preparation for this accomplishment. As anyone who has ever studied a martial art will know, it's all about the flow—and being in it. Awen?

Or maybe *The Force*? Another 20th-century mythological creation, also allied to the martial arts, and the means through which the repressive terrorism of the Empire is crushed and dismantled. Have you ever wondered why these stories are so potent and intuitive? Have you ever wondered about the machine that reproduces them as moving pictures and feeds them to us *en masse*? Are we being given the clues to our own salvation by the very means that also imprisons and enslaves us? The path to liberation in plain sight, proffered to our unseeing eyes by agents of the very forces that seek to hold us enthralled? Do these allegories hold out to us the possibility that the way to defeat the artificial, technological, suppressive, imprisoning, objectifying grids of the Matrix and the Empire is through activating the fully human, the carbon-based, organic and ensouled?

The word matrix comes from the Latin *Mater*—mother—but it can be complicated. In the film, unawakened humans gestate in a vast womb-like warehouse. On the other hand, *Pachamama*, the Earth Mother in the religion of the Inca, presides over fertility and harvest, which are thought of as the *sine qua non* of a successful culture. But as Dan Quinn's eponymous gorilla Ishmael[20] points out, the now ubiquitous and dominant agrarian cultures of our planet, cultures essentially that have reserved and enslaved certain plants and animals for the exclusive use of humans, often to the detriment of other species, have also created a singular kind of prison in which humans also languish, unknowingly, while paradoxically considering ourselves to be "free". He who controls the food supply controls the world. "Mother culture", seen in this light, is simply another facet of the Matrix.

In Quinn's formulation, the agrarian cultures are dubbed the "Takers". They take relentlessly, whatever there is to take. They are entitled, they don't stop to think about the consequences, and they have no well-developed concept of stewardship. On the other side are the "Leavers"—those who choose not to adopt the ways of the Takers; those who prefer to leave the world as it is, to tread lightly, as the saying goes, and ensure that what they use is replaced or recycled. The problem we have in our era is that the Leavers are being taken by the Takers, who do not recognise anyone's right to exist outside the system of Taking. Everyone, and everything, is given meaning and value by the gold standard of commodification and yield.

This latter situation is close indeed to the heart of one of this book's central themes: that the commodification of plants, whether for food or for medicine, or for anything else, issues from an assumption of human superiority that does not automatically apply in the natural world. Perspectivism, the theory that the knowledge of any subject is limited to the perspective of the viewer, and therefore partial and incomplete, also suggests that the perspective of the "other"—whether that be tribal, national or racial, or other orders of life (animals, plants and so forth)—is as valid as our own. In other words, the natural world is inherently non-hierarchical, or "symmetrically pluralistic"[21] We will develop this notion continuously as this book progresses.

Still, the trillion-dollar question remains unanswered: what would a new and different mindset look like? Must we all swap our sartorial pretensions for grass skirts and beads, and our stock conveniences for raw sticks and stones, and return naked and barefoot to the forest—what's left of it? Or are we, like Macbeth, "*In blood Stepped in so far that, should I wade no more, Returning were as tedious as go o'er*"?[22] In other words, folks, we might already have killed the Buddha. It looks like there's no way forward, and no way back. What the fuck?

Necessity, they say, is the mother of invention, and the necessity has never been so dire. You have heard it said, either be part of the problem, or part of the solution. But when the solutions start to repeat, proliferate and self-destruct at nauseating speed, like the insane calliopes of a bad Ayahuasca experience, what are we left with? Problems cannot be solved with the same mindset with which they were created, etc.

What we are left with is what we started with: a vibrating, oscillating field of pure energy and intention, out of which we can fashion our lives, and the world, as we would wish them to be. To apprehend the reality of this we must journey to the innermost depths of ourselves, to the point where we were induced to forget our origins, and rediscover the ways in which we are already the authors of our experience here in three dimensions. But this is an advanced solution—and it will appear the sheerest fantastical madness to most people in today's world—maybe even for some of my readers here. The problems of the world, seen macroscopically, seem too large for us as individuals. There are choices being made that far outweigh our ability to offset them—and they are after all the choices of significant numbers of others, over whom we do not have agency.

This book may be regarded as a handbook to a type of magic. I have been unable to ascertain that the etymological root of the word *magic* is the same as that for *imagination*, but it makes a kind of intuitive sense, and it is to your imagination that I wish to appeal, while also recognising that rational argument may be used to some extent to prepare the way: in other words, once you can truly understand the bind we are in, you might be ready to give something else a shot. The precise "something else" is the kernel of intention that guided me to write this book.

* * *

As I write this evening I can feel the vast and inexorable shift of the earth from summer to autumn. A fresh breeze causes me to seek out warmer clothing, and the darkening evenings drive us inside ever earlier. There is a nostalgia for the balm of Summer, and at the same time a frisson of excitement for the coming season. I love storms and weather, of all kinds. The danger of them, and the unpredictability, cause my inner landscapes to shift and stir in anticipation of new possibilities. This is one of the benefits of a life spent close to plants. Awareness of the seasons, not in a simplistic, "Oh, isn't it getting dark these days?" But a real sense of something significant, something ancient and arcane, intimations of a knowledge that might once have been the very ground upon which our ancestors stood, and into which their day to day reality, together with the skills they had developed with which to navigate it, was intricately woven.

As for contemporary herbal medicine, my field, that territory is now redolent with new techno-herbalists, using search engines, plant identification apps, online and hybrid learning, and AI-assisted research platforms. *"Our great- great-grandmothers are back,"* wrote Simon Mills and Kerry Bone in 1999. *"They may be wearing white laboratory smocks and using main-frame computers, but our great-great-grandmothers are indeed back."*[23] How uneasy is that coexistence? And should it even be happening? Is it not a complete cognitive dissonance? Have our great-great-grandmothers not in their turn been mesmerised by the jingles and sparkles of information technology? Might they too yet need to extricate themselves from the silicon-based Matrix and relearn their carbon-based craft? Might they too not need to renegotiate their initiation into the flow of Awen and Wyrd?

In terms of *medicine* the lesson of the ancients is that the healing, if that is what we seek, does not come from the drug—whether plant or chemical—any more than it comes from doctors, nurses, therapists, procedures, or any of the usual accoutrements of witch doctors and shamans—be they "indigenous" and "traditional", or the *brujos* of the modern age—the surgeons, consultants, wielders of the knife and of the peculiar magic of the pharmacological age. The healing—or the *correction*—is within us. It is not, ultimately, something we can ever step aside from, for the consequences of departure from the laws of nature are calculated to bring us back, one way or another: to realisation and health—or to death.

Notes

1. Modest Mouse. (2007). Parting of the Sensory. From *We Were Dead Before The Ship Even Sank*. Epic Records.
2. https://www.recoverysystemssport.com/pemf-impact-schumann-resonance-health/?srsltid=AfmBOoqwFmqgNPCAYKjLg5hDCbZUzfYLV9Vc5xQR8vrO-1IV5DnJzw6c.
3. https://www.sciencedirect.com/science/article/abs/pii/S1364682614001692?via%3Dihub.
4. The citation does not have academic credibility, but unofficial and unaccredited data have a habit of prefiguring what later becomes accepted theory: https://foundbyai.medium.com/what-just-happened-to-the-schumann-resonance-meditate-manifest-734ac0b7a9ea.
5. For a discussion of these effects read Buhner, S. H. (2004). *The Secret Teachings of Plants*. Rochester, VT: Bear and Company.
6. Fuller, B. (1969). *Operating Manual for Spaceship Earth*. Chapter 4. Available at: https://www.tota.world/article/2942/. Accessed 5.1.2026.
7. The boiling frog is a metaphor for slow and insidious change leading to inevitable death, in a manner that cannot be detected until it is too late.
8. Attributed to Einstein but probably made popular by Ram Dass around 1970.
9. In 1974 Henry Kissinger brokered a deal with Saudi Arabia offering military protection in exchange for their agreement to use US dollars exclusively for oil pricing and trading. Since that time, key examples of forced regime change by means of American military intervention, specifically in the Middle East and Africa, have routinely followed attempts on the part of those countries to use alternative currencies with which to trade oil. As I write this note in adding the final touches to my manuscript, the Venezuelan President, Nicolas Maduro, has been captured and is awaiting trial on charges of trafficking drugs and weapons, while the US steps in to run his country. Kissinger's petrodollar system has maintained the US as the dominant global economy in this manner for over 50 years, founded upon oil and bloodshed.
10. https://www.scientificamerican.com/article/warfares-climate-emissions-are-huge-but-uncounted/?utm_source=chatgpt.com.
11. Jackson-Main, P. (2025). *Natural Healing: Staying Well Naturally in the Modern World*. London: Aeon.
12. https://www.economist.com/business/2018/08/18/a-shock-court-verdict-against-monsantos-roundup?utm_medium=cpc.adword.

pd&utm_source=google&ppccampaignID=18156330227&ppcad ID=&utm_campaign=a.22brand_pmax&utm_content=conversion. direct-response.anonymous&gclsrc=aw.ds&gad_source=5&gad_ campaignid=18156330848&gclid=EAIaIQobChMIup_C5N-bjwMV3IKDBx1fzzwDEAAYASAAEgIzd_D_BwE.
13. Gonzalez Monserrate, S. (2022). The Cloud Is Material: On the Environmental Impacts of Computation and Data Storage. Available at: https://mit-serc.pubpub.org/pub/the-cloud-is-material/release/1.
14. Zewe, A. (2025). Explained: Generative AI's Environmental Impact. *MIT News,* available at: https://news.mit.edu/2025/explained-generative-ai-environmental-impact-0117.
15. Recke, M. (2019). *Why Imagination and Creativity are Primary Value Creators.* SinnerSchrader Aktiengesellschaft.
16. Harari, Y. N. (2015). *Sapiens: A Brief History of Humankind.* New York: HarperCollins.
17. https://www.druidry.co.uk/awen-the-holy-spirit-of-druidry/.
18. Payne, F. Anne (1974). Three aspects of Wyrd in Beowulf. *Old English Studies in Honour of John C. Pope,* ed. Robert B. Burlin and Edward B. Irving Jr. Toronto: University of Toronto Press, pp. 15–36. https://doi.org/10.3138/9781442632714-004.
19. Foucault, M. (2003). *The Birth of the Clinic.* London & New York: Routledge.
20. Quinn, D. (1992). *Ishmael.* New York: Bantam/Turner Books.
21. For a discussion of symmetrical pluralism, see McGonigle, I. V. (2017). Spirits and Molecules: Ethnopharmacology and Symmetrical Epistemological Pluralism. *Ethnos, 82*(1): 139–164.
22. Shakespeare's *Macbeth,* Act III, Scene 4.
23. Mills, S. & Bone, K. (1999). *The Principles and Practice of Phytotherapy.* London: Elsevier.

CHAPTER TWO

Exchange: a bargain with carbon

Denn alles Fleisch es ist wie Gras.

—Brahms, *Requiem*[1]

I do not intend to suggest that my personal journey with plants is any more significant or dramatic than anyone else's. Instead, I want to reawaken the memory of your own journey. Was there a time in your life when the world was magical and luminous, and contained treasures unknown waiting to be discovered? I am reaching towards something primal, resident in the deeper "childhood" of our species—perhaps to some extent still contactable in those areas of our planet where people still live close to the earth, in enduring and meaningful communion, and where the earth is still sacred and revered as the Mother, the wellspring of our physical being, and the source of our sustenance, both physical and spiritual. I refer to a time out of mind in respect of our current racial context, in which Nature has been supplanted by Culture and where the parenting of our awareness is now performed by inculcating preference, precept and prohibition, rather than by direct knowledge and apprehension. Echoes of that primal experience are, I choose to believe, present in most minds, given a little reflection and reminiscence.

Was there a time before you were taught to view plants as commodities, there for your convenience, but needing sanitisation, preparation, refinement—*cleansing* of the "filth" of Nature? Do you remember the joy of mud and slime wherein plants thrive? A deep and distant era in your life when you shared kinship with these beings as children of the Earth, and when you knew how to relate to them without having to be "taught" or instructed? Do you remember a time when their language, the language of visions, aromas and exotic tastes, was native to your own apprehension of the world? A time before you were stratified, coded, and imprinted with the signature markings of the Matrix?

Any time when you feel at peace with the world, when life feels good, when your heart bursts with the sheer joy of being alive, you are reinventing the world—*in fact*. What do you see around you in your visions? Where are you? A garden, perhaps? A favourite location "in nature"? Or do you see yourself in the office, the factory, the school, the hospital? I have no judgments about what may make you happy—happiness is to be treasured wherever it is found—but if we could take a poll of responses from this exercise I'd be willing to bet that plants are not far away for most of us in our visions of joyful remembrance, whether in the wild, cultivated, on the plate … or perhaps in a wedding bouquet?

* * *

My mother was her father's daughter when it came to plants and gardening, and she took seriously her need to pass those skills on to her children. When I was eight years old we moved to a semidetached house with a long garden, which came already divided into functional segments: the usual expanse of grass that needed constant tidying and mowing (that was my father's job—a manly, sweat-filled endeavour), bordered by shrubs and rose beds on one side and a long beech hedge on the other; a flower bed section, about which more shortly; and, behind a hedge of hawthorn with a walkway through its centre, the "wild" part of the garden, which my father tried to tame as a vegetable plot, but was predictably defeated, not because he lacked the skill or the inspiration, but due to the exigencies of his job, which involved him in almost weekly continental travel and, as befitted his senior status in the company, a fair share of late evenings in the office or the laboratory. When granted time to pursue garden activities, it was the lawn that claimed most of his attention. As a result, this was the section of the garden in which, as children, we spent most of our time. The sandpit wasn't particularly successful because the local cats had other uses for it; but the crowning glory of that end of the garden was "The Bushes", about which more below.

It was the flower beds in the middle section that my mother curated, and subdivided into three equal beds, one each for myself and my two brothers. (Our sisters were not yet born so we were "the boys".) She then had us sowing bedding plant seeds in trays of compost, germinating under glass, thinning out the seedlings and planting them out in arrangements that we were allowed to design ourselves, based on the colours available—red salvia, blue ageratum, white alyssum, yellow and orange marigold. Predictably, rivalry asserted itself very quickly, and the competition between us was keen. I could advance the theory that this was as much in respect of mother's approval as it was to do with the success of our horticultural endeavours, but it came to my attention thus that I had also apparently inherited (if one can inherit such a thing) my grandfather's gifts in the garden—at least that was my mother's explanation and interpretation as I watched in satisfied awe my plants gaining maturity, giving full realisation to my visions of colour and pattern. I was entranced by the whole process: the miracle of germination, the forceful and vigorous expression of growth, the inflamed glory of inflorescence, and the all-too-hasty capitulation to seed and die-back. I couldn't wait for the whole cycle to repeat, year on year.

Arguably more important, however, were "The Bushes" at the end of the garden, for whereas the flower-planting exercise led to rivalry and (not infrequently) fights, jealousy and tears, this dense tangle of bramble and briar at the far end of the garden was a true community resource. Tunnelling through the thicket, opening up secret passageways and establishing halls of conference and commerce, my brothers and I held sway in a space that was the envy of other kids in the neighbourhood, who despite being generously invited in on occasion, could never claim the space as their own and possessed nothing of such spectacular value in their own gardens. Moreover, of necessity, the dimensions of the labyrinth were prohibitive to adults and parents, and by reason of the thorns, far too dangerous for our sisters, when they eventually came along and begged to join in. In The Bushes we were safe, protected, inviolate—and unanimous.

* * *

It is well-known in folklore that the elder is not a tree to mess with, if you value your life and your ease. I am sheltered by one as I sit here in my garden writing, and I have learned to respect this plant. We once planted a hedge of elder along the full length of a previous garden. We enjoyed its flowers in the spring, and its berries in autumn, for several years. Then some newly arrived neighbours hacked it down one day while we were away. Horrified upon our return, we addressed the issue with them, to be told, "Strictly speaking this was on our land". Not wanting to feed the greed of lawyers, we left them to their fate. Within a year they were divorced and moved out.

You are supposed to ask permission before you touch the elder, much more taking anything from her. The terms in which you must address her are highly specific: *"Old Woman, give me some of thy wood and I will give thee some of mine when I grow into a tree"*.[2] The invocation is specifically transactional—an exchange. It is a trans-incarnational pledge. It is an inherent acknowledgment that we all borrow the accoutrements of flesh while we inhabit it, but there will come a time when we will be required, in our turn, to give it back. Elder is the guardian of the spirit world, and a psychopomp, meaning she has the power to facilitate the passage of souls to the hereafter. To know her is to understand that we cannot own even the atoms of our bodies, and we cannot take them with us. To take without due permission and attention is to invoke the consequences of disrespect—not just of the elder herself, but of the foundational terms and conditions of life in the physical. We transgress this natural law at our peril. It isn't even a matter of our carbon being stolen: the carbon was never ours in the first place.

In my energetic chart to the human iris (Figure 1), the sector containing the reflexes to the lungs is coloured green, and dubbed, "The Domain of Exchange".[3] Anatomically, referring to the lungs and their passages, we talk of the "bronchial tree", for the trachea, bronchi and bronchioles do indeed resemble, when isolated from the surrounding structures of the body, an inverted tree. The Domain of Exchange reflects not only the principle of gas exchange which takes place in the lungs, but the exchanges we conduct daily in transactions involving others, and the world at large, including what we call *love* (the fact that the heart is contained within the same domain is significant and will be discussed below). Energetic deficit in this area will highlight a need to develop responsibility along these lines, such that the individual not only fulfils his obligations in this regard but also receives the full benefit of his end of the transaction. In other words, fulfilment, including emotional fulfilment, cannot be *take* alone: it must be give *and* take.

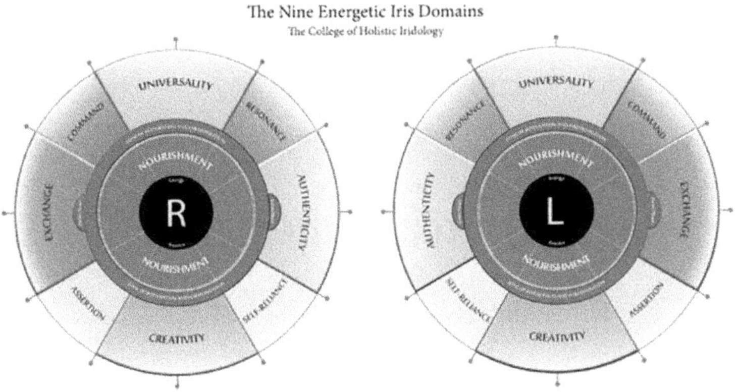

Figure 1. Energetic iris chart

Copyright © 2024. Developed by Peter Jackson-Main MSc FGNI & Anji Jackson-Main MFA. Graphics by Neterapublishing 2024.

It will not be lost on you as read this that gas exchange in the lung—carbon dioxide for oxygen—is the natural counterpart to the exchange of oxygen for carbon dioxide that is the gift of the plant world. There is one highly practical way that you can start to use this basic principle of plant metabolism, and that is through the acquisition of houseplants. In a previous volume[4] I discussed ways in which we might offset compromised and declining air quality in our time: incredibly, I forgot to mention this. I am setting that straight here. Better than electrical dehumidifiers and air-filters, houseplants can act in both capacities, while also enriching the oxygen levels in your bedroom—as well, of course, as enhancing the décor! Research conducted during the SARS-CoV-2 pandemic highlighted the possibility of using houseplants not only to ensure plentiful fresh oxygen, but also potentially to reduce transmission in enclosed spaces.[5]

But the exchange does not end there. Carbon dioxide is a vital component in the chemical equation of photosynthesis, which gives rise to *two* major products: glucose, as well as oxygen. The glucose is produced primarily for the plant itself through the mechanism of *photosynthesis* (Figure 2). It is a *primary metabolite,* which is duly circulated through the plant's vasculature for growth and proliferation (cellulose) and energy (it is used to make adenosine triphosphate, or ATP, required to power up the cells of all living organisms). Clearly, we also benefit from it when we eat plants. In fact, glucose—a basic nutrient, without which

$$6CO_2 + 6H_2O \xrightarrow{\text{Light}} C_6H_{12}O_6 + 6O_2$$

carbon dioxide — water — glucose — oxygen

Photosynthesis

Figure 2. Photosynthesis equation

we could not survive—is exclusively produced by plants and algae, both of which, of course, contain *chlorophyll.*

This substance, whose colour gives the natural world—or more specifically, the plant world—its most universally recognised signature, is a necessity for photosynthesis. The "photo" part of the word means that *light* is a part of the equation, and chlorophyll drives the process by which light (preferably sunlight) is captured and utilised by the plant. But there are further secrets in chlorophyll itself that await us in our quest to track down the intimate connections between ourselves and the world of plants. Figure 3 highlights the structural and functional properties of the molecules of chlorophyll and haemoglobin, bringing out their similar and complementary natures. It is this reciprocal functionality that enables us to talk about the "blood building" capabilities of green plants—the darker and richer the green the better—as our metabolism is able to swap out the magnesium for the iron (also contained in high amounts in green plants) to make haemoglobin, and also release the magnesium for use in regulating nerves, blood sugar, energy metabolism and much more.

Green and red, complementary colours in physics, are hardwired into the natural world as core identifiers of the vegetal and the animal respectively. But green is also the traditional colour of the heart, in energetic terms. In Indic esoteric philosophy the heart chakra, known as *Anahata* in Sanskrit, is the fourth primary energy centre in the chakra system, located at the centre of the chest. It is associated with the colour green, and when balanced and open goes towards compassion, empathy, forgiveness, love, and emotional honesty, mediating a deep sense of connection to oneself and to the world. Imbalance or constriction of the heart chakra, on the other hand, brings about isolation, mistrust, resentment, and cynicism. Cardiovascular disease, especially ischaemic

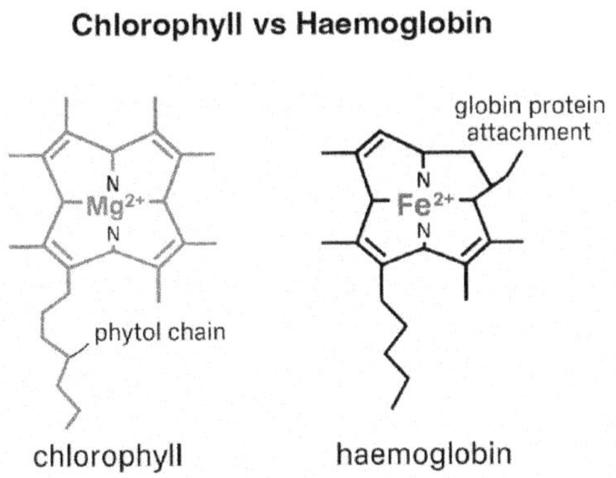

Chlorophyll	Haemoglobin
• **Core structure:** Porphyrin ring • **Central Ion:** Mg^{2}■ (Magnesium) • **Function:** Captures light for photosynthesis • **Attachment:** Phytol tail (anchors in thylakoid membranes) • **Location:** Chloroplasts (plants, algae) • **Colour:** Green pigment	• **Core structure:** Porphyrin ring • **Central Ion:** Fe^{2}■ (Iron) • **Function:** Binds and transports oxygen • **Attachment:** Globin protein (forms haemoglobin) • **Location:** Red blood cells (animals) • **Colour:** Red pigment

Figure 3. Chlorophyll and haemoglobin

circulatory disease, results in the cutting-off of the life blood to the heart itself and is the physical counterpart of energetic depletion in terms of lack of social connection, emotional warmth, and familial love and care.

I have discussed the energetics of the heart in depth in my previous volume, *The Mind's Eye*. Physiologically the heart is also involved in supporting the parasympathetic nerve response, partly by actively balancing out the neuroendocrine chemistry of the sympathetic nerve response by selective secretion of modulatory hormones.[6] Energetically and emotionally, heart-centred awareness goes towards community, companionship, collaboration and compassion, and stands in functional opposition (or counterbalance) to the biochemistry of the hypothalamic–pituitary–adrenal system, which prepares us for survival in the face of danger by emphasising competition, combat and capitulation to the ultimata of authority, and which, although to some extent biologically necessary, has been rendered the pathological default setting for many human beings in the contemporary cultural context.

We can very easily see the ways in which this basic human physiology has been hijacked and exploited by our political and corporate sectors. We are sold things we can easily do without by being convinced that NOT having them will render us vulnerable. We are convinced by our political, propagandist and advertorial puppet-masters, for example, that such-and-such a person, social group, political party, nation, race, is a poisonous enemy and must be resisted, avoided, neutralised, destroyed at all costs. This is also rolled out into the "natural" world: such-and-such a plant, animal or insect pest, virus or bacterium, must be chemically destroyed in order that we may be safe. And we don't argue—most of us. We buy the remedy, whatever it happens to be, whatever it might cost—our vote, our allegiance, our financial power (such as it is), our support for wars of all kinds, including those on "disease"—ANTI-biotics (anti-life), all kinds of allopathic (suppressive) medications, and, last but not least "immunisations". To be immune—what's not to like? But are we ever? If you have been paying attention you will have started to doubt this as a direct result of our very recent epidemiological history: one vaccination, two vaccinations, are not enough. You need regular boosters, and when you have had these, another "new variant" of the virus will inevitably be announced, which is not covered by your last booster, so, guess what …

The nature of these kinds of exchanges, these bargains that we make with those who present themselves as our saviours, is bogus. In fact, they are not true exchanges at all. They are a form of robbery. We are being grifted every which way we look. No matter what solutions we buy into, political, financial or medical, there is always something else that will come in and need "dealing with". And then, guess who will be there to offer us the "solution"? (*Ker-ching.*)

This is why we are continuously warned not to place our faith in "untested" remedies, for which no "evidence" of effectiveness is forthcoming. Even if it were, the guardians of the evidence stakes have ensured that they have legislated for that by creating the *hierarchy of evidence*, in which all forms of evidence are not equal.[7] Again, they are acting to protect us, aren't they? From what? From the quacks and the charlatans who would have you believe that taking plant medicine is a viable choice for health and vitality, for example? From people, let's face it, like me. They are simply trying to prevail against the competition: it's a basic biological imperative, isn't it?

Well, that's a matter of dispute too. The narrative of evolution, as outlined in Darwin's *Origin of Species*, ostensibly emphasises "survival of the fittest". Can you see how that story, our most era-defining creation myth, gave birth to a pantheon of theorists, including Jacques Monod's mechanistic *Chance and Necessity*,[8] and Richard Dawkins'

The Selfish Gene,[9] and the assumed supremacy of "scientific enquiry" over any other modality of perceiving and apprehending the world? But as Bruce Lipton reminds us, there was an early contemporary of Darwin who thought things through very differently. Jean-Baptiste Lamarck (1744–1829), he notes, "*suggested that evolution was based on an 'instructive', cooperative interaction among organisms and their environment that enables life forms to survive and evolve in a dynamic world*".[10] In other words, an ethics of complexity, co-operation and copoiesis, not of competition, consumption and co-option.

Even in terms of "the evidence", however, therapeutic interventions for healing the heart, physically, emotionally and energetically, through visual exposure to and immersion in the green of nature, have been shown to reduce stress, lower blood pressure and promote feelings of calm and emotional stability. Time spent in proximity to plants, sometimes referred to as "green therapy" or "forest bathing", is associated with clinically significant improvements in mental clarity, mood, cardiovascular health and immune function. Physiologically, green surroundings encourage relaxation of the central and autonomic nerve systems, while psychologically they nurture feelings of hope, compassion and connection.[11,12]

An interesting consequence of elevated carbon levels is a significant increase in the greening of the planet, with carbon fertilisation thought to be the biggest driver.[13] Not wishing to labour the point as to whether the climate science is "settled", the consensus has always had its detractors. Among the most recent, Richard Lindzen, Professor of Earth, Atmospheric, and Planetary Sciences, Emeritus, Massachusetts Institute of Technology, and William Happer, Professor of Physics, Emeritus, Princeton University, argue with conviction that, "*More carbon dioxide will create more food,*" while also demonstrating that the warming effect of increasing CO_2 levels is algorithmically limited: "*CO_2 … becomes a less effective greenhouse gas at higher concentrations because of what in physics is called 'saturation.' Each additional increase of CO_2 in the atmosphere causes a smaller and smaller change in 'radiative forcing,' or in temperature.*"[14]

Predictably the paper was widely condemned by a posse of political and scientific commentators, but much of the criticism was directed towards the "emeritus" status of the authors, with a few contributors commenting that the professors were too old to have significant views on the matter.[15] (I mention the fact only to highlight the irresponsibility of using an *ad hominem* argument in rebuttal of a carefully reasoned position.) But aside from any impact on global warming, the obvious fact that plants, at least, will benefit from higher levels of atmospheric CO_2 is not disputed. It also brings into view the overlapping impact of deforestation and desertification, especially that of the Amazon rainforest. It is estimated that a whopping 20% of the Brazilian rainforest has already gone, and although there are signs of a slow-down in the rate of deforestation, and many strenuous campaigns seem to be making headway in this, it has also been estimated that should that figure reach 40%, we may face the possibility of collapse of the entire forest system.

The Amazon rainforest is estimated to absorb a quarter of all CO_2 absorbed by all the land on earth, but its capacity has reduced by 30% within the last 35 years owing to deforestation. Loss of this vital resource could prove catastrophic and is a known contributory factor to climate change parameters. It also results in the loss of carbon sink and the release of huge amounts of extra carbon into the atmosphere.

The regreening of the earth would seem, then to be something of an urgent necessity. Hence perhaps, once more, an invitation to rethink the suppressive intervention of "net zero", as also to consider some extreme outliers in terms of ecological and evolutionary modelling? Maybe the earth already has its own remedy for these eventualities? Maybe increased carbon is part of that? Dai Ato, an independent Japanese researcher, presents data that suggests that oceanic carbon release, independent of human activity, is the true determinant of atmospheric CO_2 levels, and concludes, *"This result indicates that human efforts to curb CO_2 emissions have been, at least in the past, meaningless."*[16] Oh dear. So what now? *"You're gonna run to the sea, but the sea will be boiling."*[17]

A new look at all this might start by upending our usual conception of ourselves as the highest form of agency on the planet. Humans usually regard themselves as independent agents, uniquely capable of invention and control, and with technology as our crowning achievement and indisputable evidence of our superiority, as of our distinctiveness from the rest of life. When we "domesticate" other species, plants and animals, we rarely stop to consider whether in fact the boot may be surreptitiously on the other foot. In binding ourselves to agricultural food species, for example, are we not also potentially being used by them as their preferred method of propagation and survival?

The foundation of our belief in our own supremacy is literally biblical. In Genesis we are told that "God" (or whomever is referred to by the plural pronoun in this passage) gave us dominion over all these species: *"Let us make mankind in our image, in our likeness, so that they may rule over the fish in the sea and the birds in the sky, over the livestock and all the wild animals, and over all the creatures that move along the ground."*[18] Equally, of course, the theory of evolution itself clearly implies that we are the summit of the pyramid, the most advanced species to have been thrown up so far in the evolutionary project. Or does it? Apparently, it does not. Even in Darwin's model, natural selection merely ensures that traits that improve survival and reproduction in a given environment get passed on. It doesn't aim for "progress" or a "final form". There is no evolutionary ladder with humans at the top. In that sense, humans are not "more evolved" than bacteria or oak trees—we are just differently adapted. Most of us, however, unwittingly sign up to the biblical, rather than the scientific, narrative—which is odd given that religious fundamentalism of the old order is reportedly a minority pursuit in these days of the new fundamentalism of hard-headed scientism.[19]

Merlin Sheldrake's book, *Entangled Life,* is a richly illustrated deep-dive into the world of fungi. Sheldrake frames fungi as master influencers.[20] He delves into the ecosystem that he terms the "Wood Wide Web", in which fungal systems interact determinately with plant species in the provision of goods, services and exchanges that directly mirror (or perhaps serve as the original model for) human-devised methods of trade and commerce. The economy is precisely and minutely monitored and administered, and takes place with a clear baseline of mutual benefit and interdependency.

Sheldrake goes further. Reaching into the human realm, yeasts co-created bread, beer and wine, profoundly influencing the shape of human settlements and rituals, and thus ensuring their continuing value in cultivation. Psychoactive fungal species catalyse spiritual and cultural practices and potentially impact on human consciousness itself in ways that ensure deep commitment to returning usage—as also perhaps in enhanced reverence and regard for the sanctity of Nature. Medicinal mushrooms shape systems of healing—not just in traditional medicine, but in contemporary approaches to cancer and other pathologies which our current pharmaceutical system struggles to fully encompass. In cultivating fungi, we spread their spores and ensure their survival in a mutual project of domestication in action.

It does not take a huge leap of imagination to allow for a similar symbiotic relationship between humankind and plants. Most, however, before they have thought about it, will not take that to the next level and recognise a space in our rational evaluation for the notion that plants and fungi may also embody consciousness or agency. To say that "Nature" has devised a system of mutual co-operation and co-dependency is one thing: to grant intentionality to the non-human components in that system is still somewhat outside our current ontological and epistemological reach. Animism, the perception that all things have spirit, agency and free will, is regarded not just as a quaint-but-obsolete metaphysics, but an inherent descriptor of a *primitive* cultural orientation.

However, Sheldrake, through his father, Rupert, was party to a world-view that comes close to reestablishing such ideas as valid, and congruent with the evidence. Sheldrake senior was the originator of the concept of *Morphic Resonance*,[21] a bold and inclusive vision of reality which suggests that the "habits" of an evolving universe are stored in organised, organismic structures of consciousness called morphic fields. Along with British scientist James Lovelock, creator of the Gaia hypothesis, which proposes that the earth and its biosphere constitute a coherent, dynamic, intelligent and interdependent system, Sheldrake has been the harbinger (although as we might expect not universally accepted) of a movement that aims to rescue the natural sciences from their current mechanistic, human-centred epistemic straitjacket, and restructure our perception of the world we inhabit along more widely democratic principles, affirming agency as endemic throughout creation—which seems to define a system as close to animism as it is possible to get in contemporary terms. Michael Ellis Green claims that both Lovelock and Sheldrake are effective co-conspirators with quantum physicist David Bohm:

> *... who proposes that mind and matter both arise from the "Implicate Order," a realm of "undivided wholeness" that underlies and interconnects everything in the physical universe. These theories can be integrated: the implicate order underlies the universe, manifesting as morphic fields of causative intelligence which coordinate all activities within the universe, including those of Gaia. The universe is pervaded by intelligence and creativity, and within its structures, human mental activity is interactive and causative. If these theories are proved valid, non-local and causative mental phenomena have a scientific basis.*[22]

In a previous book, *The Mind's Eye*, I referred to the new research field of Quantum Biology, invoking it for its ability to validate a quantum approach to the necessary intersection and interdependency of mind and matter in a biological context.

Donna Jeanne Haraway, American Professor Emerita in feminist studies and the history of consciousness, is also deeply critical of the anthropocentric narratives that drive our culture. Preferring to designate our era the *Chthulucene*,[23] rather than the *Anthropocene*, her book *Staying with the Trouble* emphasises sympoiesis ("making together") over the assumption of autopoietic construction of the world by humans.[24] However, the significance of her project also reaches (some might note alarmingly) into concerns voiced in Chapter 1 about the role and agency of machines. In *A Cyborg Manifesto*,[25] Haraway rejects the rigid categories of "human", "animal" and "machine" and argues that the boundaries between them are increasingly blurred. A "cyborg" is not just a sci-fi hybrid, but a metaphor for how we live: bodies interwoven in tentacular complexity with technologies (pacemakers, prosthetics, computers, smartphones, household gadgets, personal and public transport systems, and so forth). She rejects the myth of humans as separate, pure, or "natural." Instead, we are all cyborgs—that is, we are hybrids, already technologised and without secure boundaries upon which to rely in asserting our individual "identity". Remember the question from Chapter 1: does Awen flow through machines? It appears that it might indeed do so, by virtue of their relationship with us.

Peter K. Haff, Professor Emeritus of Biology, proposes the related concept of the *Technosphere*, which he notes is *"the defining structure of the Anthropocene"*, and which is *"undesigned, autonomous and possesses agency"*.[26] He also notes that it is a significant competitor for energy, and warns of its fundamental unsustainability, which also makes the point that the greatest danger of the Technosphere is its autonomy: it appears no longer to be under our control. The fundamental question and principle of exchange goes begging once we realise that we may have created a monster that will very probably continue along a path of ever-increasing consumption, and there may be little we can do to stop it.

The question of non-human agency is a major theme of this book, and from the perspective of plant medicine it is echoed in the work of my colleague, Guy Waddell, in his book, *The Enchantment of Western Herbal Medicine*.[27] Waddell suggests that we might view the relationship between humans and plants as that of each-others' "convivial tools"—an expression borrowed from social philosopher Ivan Illich.[28] The notion of conviviality (*living with* each other in a fundamentally friendly and jovial manner) elicits images of an easy give and take. Illich himself, writing in 1973, somewhat ahead of the crisis that we now see looming, raised the possibility that we may indeed have "convivial" relationships with our tools, but that we need at all costs to maintain control over our own energy and limit our use of such tools responsibly. It begs the question, can we ever have that kind of relationship with a tool that is exercising its autonomy in the way that we see, and that Haff describes, in the Technosphere? And what kind of equal exchange is possible in that scenario—if any?

* * *

The evening pushes further into Autumn, with darkness descending in a sudden veil as my attention is drawn into these matters. The day has brought intermittent rain showers and an uneasy wind. I reflect that my own chthonic partner and convivial tool, the redoubtable MacBook Pro, has not yet mastered adaptation to water, and so I had to relocate several times to within the garden studio from the small patio under our canopy of companion trees. I am still wearing shorts and sandals. I haven't caught up yet. Writing about Nature is not the same as being in it. Stiff and cold, I rise to take the winding path back to the house.

Intuitively, I feel a danger lurking in these hypothetical regions. It is not necessarily inherent in the specific properties of machines. It is scarcely conceivable that we can live on this planet in our present numbers without technology to assist us in administering our most urgent needs. But the danger is that machinery itself, as a product of capitalism, is resolutely oligarchic in origin, in realisation, and in perpetuation. It is not offered to the world as a contribution: it is sold to us in exchange not only for money, but for our obeisance and the loss of our self-determination. It is the difference between the transformative vision of Nikola Tesla in seeking to bring wireless energy to the world, and the entrepreneurial overreach of Elon Musk in exploiting the invention of the electric vehicle in making himself the richest individual human on the planet. It is the difference between the old-style mechanical vehicles that one could (and I regularly did) dismantle and service inside out with the aid of the relevant Haynes Manual, and the new computer-dependent, mechanically locked contraptions that demand dealership involvement, or at the very least, state of the art service stations. *Ker-ching.*

Again, problems cannot be solved with the same mindset that created them. It is not that we may have to make space for machines and technology in a communal environment: it is that the politics and economics of technology do not, at present, belong to us equally. Put simply, the *exchange* value of such things is heavily weighted towards the self-interest of the entrepreneurs (who are not even necessarily the inventors, but simply those who have made it their business to promote and therefore profit from them). And while we may, in the short term, benefit from them (their role in facilitating this book has been noted), in the long term we may pay a dear price. Unless we can find a way to liberate the machines themselves from their own exploitation in the capitalist drama, perhaps?

So, where are plants in all this? These too are companion species with whom we have been entangled for millennia, aeons even. And yet still, despite all that they offer us, we scarcely offer them a second thought in thinking through and deciding our experimental futures—other than to commodify them as "food" or "building materials", or "textiles" or even as "the lungs of the earth". Are these beings disadvantaged and disenfranchised in this equation, or are they, unbeknownst to us, quietly waiting their turn, unruffled and unconcerned as we thrash about in our ontological quagmire of linguistic nonsense?

This chapter has brought forward the principle of exchange—the fundamental economy of the natural world. Clever intellectual notions such as sympoiesis and symbiosis are utterly dependent upon it. And the beautiful truth of this is that, even if we don't pay attention, and we don't consciously fulfil our part of the bargain, even if we leave out whole swathes of creation in our resolute focus upon our own visible advantages and benefits, sooner or later we will be subject to its laws. We will find that we cannot but return what we owe. *Somehow, someone else will steal your carbon.* Once again, the plants know the truth of this. All they need do is wait.

Notes

1. English tr. "For all flesh is as grass". The text for Brahms' Requiem is adapted from Isaiah 40, 6–8.
2. https://druidry.org/druid-way/teaching-and-practice/druid-tree-lore/elder.
3. See Jackson-Main, P. (2024). *The Mind's Eye: Personality and Behaviour as Revealed in Quantum Iris Analysis*. London: Aeon.

4. Jackson-Main, P. (2025). *Natural Healing: Staying Well Naturally in the Modern World*. London: Aeon.
5. El-Tanbouly, R., Hassan, Z., El-Messeiry, S. (2021). The Role of Indoor Plants in Air Purification and Human Health in the Context of COVID-19 Pandemic: A Proposal for a Novel Line of Inquiry. *Frontiers in Molecular Biosciences, 30*(8): 709395. doi: 10.3389/fmolb.2021.709395. PMID: 34277711; PMCID: PMC8279815.
6. See Buhner, S. H. (2004). *The Secret Teachings of Plants in the Direct Perception of Nature*. London: Aeon, pp. 78–82.
7. In medical terms, the hierarchy of evidence prioritises meta reviews and RCTs (randomised, double-blinded, placebo-controlled trials). But these are precisely chosen to assess certain types of medical interventions, particularly pharmaceuticals. There is nothing wrong, *per se*, with selecting an evidence type to answer the specific research question that you have; but the problem is that the elevation of this kind of research has become an absolute in evidence terms, such that modalities that are very poorly and inadequately served by them are nonetheless required to submit themselves to the presumed authority of the dominant methodology.
8. Monod, J. (1974). *Chance and Necessity*. New York: HarperCollins.
9. Dawkins, R. (2016). *The Selfish Gene*. Oxford: Oxford University Press.
10. Lipton, B. (2015). *The Biology of Belief: Unleashing the Power of Consciousness*. London: Hay House, p. 42.
11. Wen, Y., Yan, Q., Pan, Y. et al. (2019). Medical Empirical Research on Forest Bathing (*Shinrin-yoku*): A Systematic Review. *Environmental Health and Preventive Medicine, 24*: 70. https://doi.org/10.1186/s12199-019-0822-8.
12. Hunter, M., Gillespie, B., Chen, S. (2019). Urban Nature Experiences Reduce Stress in the Context of Daily Life Based on Salivary Biomarkers. *Frontiers in Psychology*, 10. https://doi.org/10.3389/fpsyg.2019.00722.
13. Gui, Y., Wang, K., Huntingford, C. et al. (2025). Vegetation Greenness in 2024. *Nature Reviews Earth & Environment, 6*: 255–257. https://doi.org/10.1038/s43017-025-00656-z.
14. https://co2coalition.org/wp-content/uploads/2025/06/Lindzen-Happer-GHGs-and-Fossil-Fuels-Climate-Physics-2025-06-07.pdf.
15. https://skepticalscience.com/search.php?t=c&Search=Will+Happer.
16. Ato, D. (2024). *Multivariate Analysis Rejects the Theory of Human-caused Atmospheric Carbon Dioxide Increase: The Sea Surface Temperature Rules*. Independent researcher, Osaka, Japan. Available at: https://

scienceofclimatechange.org/wp-content/uploads/SCC-Ato-Multivariate-Analysis-Vol.4.2.pdf.
17. Peter Tosh. (1977). Downpressor man. *Equal Rights*. Columbia Records.
18. Genesis 1, New International Version, available at: https://www.biblegateway.com/passage/?search=Genesis%201&version=NIV.
19. In citing evolutionary theory, by the way, I am not pledging full support for that theory, as will become obvious as you read further.
20. Sheldrake, M. (2020). *Entangled Life: How Fungi Make Our Worlds, Change Our Minds and Shape Our Futures*. London: The Bodley Head.
21. Sheldrake, R. (2009). *Morphic Resonance: The Nature of Formative Causation*. Rochester, VT: Park Street Press.
22. Green, M. E. (1998). *Visions of Unity: An Exploration of the Scientific Theories of James Lovelock and Rupert Sheldrake*. Florida State University. Available at: https://philpapers.org/rec/GREVOU.
23. The term "Chthulucene" was coined by Donna Haraway and is derived from the Greek words "chthon" (meaning "earth" or "underworld") with the suffix "-cene" denoting a geological era.
24. Haraway, D. J. (2016). *Staying with the Trouble: Making Kin in the Chthulucene*. Durham, NC: Duke University Press.
25. Haraway, D. J. (1991). A Cyborg Manifesto: Science, Technology, and Socialist-Feminism in the Late Twentieth Century. In her *Simians, Cyborgs and Women: The Reinvention of Nature*. New York: Routledge, pp. 149–181.
26. Haff, P. K. (2023). "Technosphere". In Nathanaël Wallenhorst & Christoph Wulf, *Handbook of the Anthropocene*. Cham: Springer Verlag, pp. 537–541. Available at: https://philarchive.org/rec/HAFTXX. Accessed 4.1.2026.
27. Waddell, G. (2020). *The Enchantment of Western Herbal Medicine: Herbalists, Plants, and Nonhuman Agency*. London: Aeon.
28. Illich, I. (2021). *Tools for Conviviality*. Delhi: Aakar Books.

CHAPTER THREE

The nature of Nature

Redeveloping the capacity for heart-centred cognition can help each of us reclaim personal perception of the living and sacred intelligence within the world, within each particular thing. It moves us from a rational orientation in a dead, mechanised universe to one in which the unique perceptions of the heart are noticed and strengthened, to a deep experience of the living soulfulness of the world.

Stephen Harrod Buhner[1]

Those who have spent any time on the land working to bring forth its bounty, whether in comestible produce or dazzling aesthesis, will know that it is a task without end. One must give up the idea of "finishing the job" in favour of an exacting and perpetual servitude to the sheer aggressive, thrusting vitality of plants. The most lovingly manicured garden, if left untended for even a few days, will very quickly start to appear at first slightly ragged, then distinctly overgrown, before becoming, in the space of only a few weeks, a complex wilderness of competing populations of plants, as they try to extricate themselves from the grid imposed upon them by humans and establish their own order.

I remember a popular walk that I used to take on the outskirts of the Surrey town in which I grew up. Visiting a friend just around the corner in a quiet residential close, we frequently ventured up the local road from which the close diverged, passing about a half-mile series of secluded, well-appointed houses, which gave way in due course to an even less dense stratum of human habitation—country cottages and smallholdings—before entering a region of woodland. At this stage the metalled road started to fragment and crumble at the edges, developing a central ridge of weed growth where the wheels of now very occasional vehicles did not encroach. The track, as it had now become, before disappearing completely into meadow and a rough footpath (now intersected by the M23 motorway), veered sharply right at a certain point, and then left, as it circumnavigated an impenetrable density of trees and undergrowth, which a local map gave us to understand was the site of a small motte and bailey construction dating back to Norman times.[2] It was impossible for us to verify this assertion, although we intrepidly fought our way through the tangle of bough and brushwood to apprehend the murky semblance of a mound surrounded by a vaguely defined ditch and thick with wild growth. The ditch impossible to cross; the mound inaccessible; whatever went before now long gone; a palimpsest of plant agency.

The fate that awaits buildings if no one inhabits or tends to them is more than simply dereliction. Human constructions are maintained by human intention. Otherwise, they fall prey to other intentions, and plants are particularly skilled at destroying buildings, as is evident in the story of the outlawing of Japanese knotweed as a garden plant in the UK. *Fallopia japonica* is in fact a redoubtable plant medicine for its ability to break down hard structures within the body, including cysts and cancerous tumours, which seems to provide a functional echo to its "nuisance" value as a noxious and invasive "weed" capable of destroying buildings. A form of existential chemotherapy, perhaps?

There is something intensely congruous about this. In homeopathy, the cancer miasm[3] has been described as embodying feelings of being trapped, restricted, overburdened by duty, or unable to reconcile inner needs with outer expectations; a life lived under compartmentalisation, conforming outwardly while inwardly feeling helpless, divided and full of unexpressed rage and frustration. The tumour represents the repressed emotional energy of resistance and self-assertion. We might note echoes with the taming and homogenisation of nature itself in large-scale agricultural projects, forestry management, and horticulture. Humans always seem to want to put things in grids and in boxes—including ourselves.

Nevertheless, it was in a well-tended garden, with scintillating rockeries, sweeping borders, arboreal shelters, a swathe of green velvet lawn, and a picturesque riverside sedge, that one of my most important and constitutional epiphanies took place. The garden belonged to a house owned by a now long-collapsed initiative in my home city. The Cambridge Centre was conceived and run as a community resource space for meditation, philosophy and spiritual practices, healing and education. The Centre activities themselves were delivered from more central premises in Cambridge City, but the house, bordering the river on the outskirts of the historic city centre, while still within the city limits, had been gifted to the Centre by a benefactor—sadly at this distance in time I have forgotten who, and since this was all a few years in advance of the internet, it has proved impossible to retrieve the history of this once signature local initiative in alternative living. If any readers are able to fill in the gaps I would delight in hearing from them.

City centre premises, even at that era, were expensive to maintain, and so the fate of the property (which obviously still exists, and whose garden may still be viewed from the appropriate vantage point) was to be put on the market—effectively cannibalised to keep the "Centre" going. It was not a popular decision. Even at that era I was savvy enough to know that you do not exchange real estate that you own outright for the ability to pay rent on a property that does not belong to you—especially not without a good business plan, and there was nothing of the kind—and I said so. But I, along with others, were sadly outvoted by the trustees. I am on that account extra thankful that the opportunity that came my way in the garden was made temporarily possible within that timeline.

One day in the early summer of 1992 a party was thrown for supporters of the Centre in the garden of this property. A light shower of summer rain had left the grass and the rockery plants glistening with rainbow drops, reflecting shards of light that played on the back of my retina (or was that the effect of the champagne?). Someone was asking me what I did, and what my plans were. I had recently been made forcibly redundant from an employment that had ended in rancour and legal action, and I was "between opportunities", as they say. I remember being aware of a curious force arising inside of me, something to which I had to give utterance. Gesturing broadly towards the rockery, I found myself suddenly eloquent in extolling the bounty of nature in providing for all our needs, and I announced, formally and with authority, my full intention to make the study of herbal medicine my next major project.

I mentioned that there was to be a course in Spain in November with the renowned Dr Richard Schulze, and that I was somehow determined to be there. I did not know how I was going to afford it but was certain that some miracle would intervene to make it possible. My one-person audience simply said, cryptically, "I think we can do a bit better than that". I had no idea what she meant and did not give it another thought, until I received a message, a few days later, requesting my bank details.

> *Whatever you can do, or dream you can, begin it*
> *Boldness has genius, power, and magic in it.*[4]

It would be fanciful, of course, to claim that the plants were in any way responsible for this epiphany. Wouldn't it? You see, after over three decades as a herbalist, I am as certain as I can be that plants both listen and respond to our deepest wishes and intentions. The magic of the moment—amplified by the champagne (yeasts in action once more)—was a unifying experience, in which I was temporarily colonised by an initiative that seemed to originate quite outside of my usual habits of thought and speech. For a start, I was rarely at that era quite so decisive in "real life", preferring to downplay my expectations and intentions with faux humility, rather than release impossibly large ideas upon the world—even though I might harbour them. In that moment, it seemed, "something" took over. Was I "channelling" the plants? Something else? But I clearly remember the surprise that I experienced in hearing myself utter those words—a surprise that was redoubled when the money I needed to follow through arrived in my bank account a few days later.

* * *

The universe that perpetually invents itself. A multifaceted, ever-changing symbol of everything—*All That Is*. I prefer the concept of *immanence* to the usually accepted *transcendence* when it comes to the discussion of the numinous or spiritual dimensions of life. To transcend is to go beyond, or outside of a system. But how can you go outside of reality? Just because we do not see all of reality, does not exclude that those parts that are outside of our field of awareness are nonetheless inherent parts of the system. It's the same with the word "supernatural": how can anything be *super*-natural—*above* what is natural?

Surely, it's all just … natural? Likewise, the term "universe" does not need to disambiguated by reference to a "multiverse"—an attempt to cater for the possibility that there may be more than one system. Surely the *universe* comprises all possible systems? The clue is in the name—"UNI-verse".

Immanence—the idea that the divine (energy) encompasses or is manifested within the material world—can apply to both monotheistic and pantheistic systems of spiritual or religious thought. Everything is in God, and God is in everything. Everything IS God, and God IS everything. Why is this important?

We do not simply parachute into a mechanistic world that we then manipulate in ways that happen to serve us. We are not just visitors here. We create ourselves, and we create our worlds. We make our lives, our environments, the conditions that we find, the encounters that we need. And, with our direct co-operation, the world constantly creates and recreates itself as a multipartite system that layers levels of consciousness throughout its constituents, from the micro to the macro: from subatomic particles and units of energy, right up to supermassive black holes and the galaxies that they drive. We are all part of That, and That is part of us. The strong anthropic principle in physics suggests that a universe without witnesses is an impossibility. We might rephrase that to suggest that witnesses are constitutional, and generative, for the universe.

That may be why pantheistic and *panpsychic* systems, after all, may serve us better in the quest to understand the nature of the universe—the nature of Nature itself. If each component part of the whole has, to its own extent and character, consciousness and agency, then the entire thing is zinging with energy and determination, and a fundamental creative intelligence that leaves no part of itself untouched and unappointed.

Haraway's sympoiesis gives way to copoiesis in this vision. We exist in a magnificent collaborative construct, and our co-creators are everywhere around us: fellow humans, for sure, but other orders of life—plants, animals, fungi, bacteria, etc. We recruit even the basic building blocks of reality through persuasion to mutually beneficial ends, with which to create our intimate physical forms. Within these forms exist many other self-determined species. It has been estimated that although the content by volume and mass of our physical bodies is more than 99% "our own", the content in terms of the number of cells that do not "belong" to us is around 56% in bacterial microbiota.[5] In other words, although these denizens of our bodies only weigh approximately 0.2 kg, they actually outnumber our own cells, numerically. And they have well-defined roles to play in regulating our physiology *and* our psychology. That's a whole lot of collaborators and co-creators right there.

Even if we talk about "our own" cells in this equation, as Bruce Lipton reminds us, our purported evolution into multicellular organisms was in effect a project of collaborative, co-operative self-interest among participating cells, the idea being the survival advantage—strength in numbers.[6] Lipton's vision of our bodies as an aggregate of co-operating cells, each with their own nucleus (and therefore their own "brain", and putatively, their own self-determination) is fully resonant with the vision of a universe composed of multiple consciousnesses, or we might say, multiple focal points of awareness, collaborating in a shared construction. Our bodies themselves are the product of a shared construction.

The idea of a perpetually self-creating universe has begun to enter scientific discourse and challenges the notion of a singular beginning point in the far distant past, leading to a mechanistic set of consequences that although complex, are still essentially predictable. Instead, the idea of the universe as an autopoietic process, a living intelligence continually producing and sustaining itself, recommends itself to our present enquiry and has gained a certain amount of ground at the margins of science—we referred in the previous chapter to the contributions of Lovelock, Sheldrake and Bohm. The term *autopoiesis* itself was coined in 1980 by biologists Humberto Maturana and Francisco Varela, to refer to the self-production that defines living systems.[7] Their analysis interestingly can be applied to both macroscopic and microscopic living systems, from a single cell to a whole community or environment.

Varela a little later (1992) collaborated with professor of philosophy Evan Thompson and psychologist Eleanor Rosch in the development of theory that they termed *enactivism*,[8] which holds that

> *the species brings forth and specifies its own domain of problems … this domain does not exist 'out there' in an environment that acts as a landing pad for organisms that somehow drop or parachute into the world. Instead, living beings and their environments stand in relation to each other through mutual specification or codetermination.*[9]

And again,

> *Organisms do not passively receive information from their environments, which they then translate into internal representations. Natural cognitive systems ... participate in the generation of meaning ... engaging in transformational and not merely informational interactions:* they enact a world.[10]

The fact that these ideas have not generated significant traction in mainstream natural sciences probably owes itself to that fact that they come dangerously close to an expression of *panpsychism*—a longstanding philosophical orientation that was supposedly displaced in the early 20th century by the arrival of logical positivism. Logical positivism aspired to an empirically demonstrable and verifiable set of philosophical operations—a philosophical facsimile of empirical science perhaps. In doing so it necessarily pronounced metaphysics, theology and ethics meaningless. It was itself doomed to collapse under the weight of the science it so cravenly tried to emulate, attracting criticism, notably, from both Karl Popper and Thomas Kuhn, themselves key commentators on the philosophy of science.[11]

The antecedents of panpsychism, however, as a European philosophical system, go back at least as far Plato and include Spinoza, Leibnitz, Schopenhauer and, more recently, Bertrand Russell. Contemporary defences of the idea can be found among "philosophers of mind" Kastrup,[12] Goff[13] and Mathews,[14] who suggest that, far from being a blindly mechanistic phenomenon, the universe is in fact a "mind-saturated" process. The cosmos is consciousness in action, and each of us is a locally differentiated portion of that larger intelligence.

The reawakening of interest in these ideas has also followed, or in some cases has been contemporaneous with, the arrival of esoterically derived material that has affirmed very similar, if not identical premises. The phrase *All That Is*, now something of a commonplace in metaphysical discourses as a descriptive epithet for God, was first brought to the world in the writings of American psychic Jane Roberts, who between 1963 and her death in 1984 channelled an "off-world" entity who announced himself as *Seth*. Seth describes himself as *"an energy essence no longer focussed in physical reality"*[15] and presents a cosmology that has lit up the imaginations of countless readers and thinkers, including doctors, scientists, healers, artists, writers and philosophers.

Seth's metaphysics rests on the following principles: 1. Reality is first and foremost psychological—mind creates matter, not the other way around, and ALL matter possesses consciousness, down to the smallest particle. 2. Mind itself is a production of our energy essence, or soul; we are each the authors our own reality, through the agency of consciousness, and each one of us is "eternally valid" and fundamentally indestructible. 3. *All That Is* contains everything, and every possible or probable variation on everything, and perpetually infuses its creations with its own abundant creative energy. 4. Time is not linear, but simultaneous, and the fulcrum of the power to "hack" the system and make changes in our lives is to enter fully into the present moment.

The books are more than philosophical or metaphysical tracts: they are also highly practical manuals for living as co-operating participants in a vast, self-producing, intelligent, blazingly conscious system of reality. Seth's propositions are regarded as foundational in these terms, and although a few similar texts have been produced in recent times, none have quite so eloquently, vividly and *joyfully* expounded the nature of the system of reality that we inhabit as these revelatory transmissions from the latter half of the 20th century.

However, even in these examples there is relatively little commentary on plants as collaborators in our world. For that we need to go to different sources, and enter the realms of anthropology and ethnobotany, in particular, studies of the Amerindian populations of North, Central and South America. It is here, particularly in South America and most specifically in the Amazon rainforest, that we find a cosmology that admits and includes plants alongside humans as co-conspirators in the production of reality. The use of the so-called "Master Plants" in this geographical area, some of which have strong psychoactive effects, is something that I will address a little later on in this book, but it is worth pointing out that the plants themselves in these traditions are considered directly responsible for the knowledge held about them: in other words, the answer to the question, how did these people know so much about the plants in their environment is: *they learned directly from the plants themselves*. Compare that with the way in which the civilised, Europeanised world objectifies and dissects its environment and its cohabiting species—and even the human itself—in the effort to describe and reveal them, and it is fully obvious that entirely different epistemic and phenomenological regimes operate in these traditional and aboriginal human populations.

As ever, the lay thinker must exercise restraint and caution in approaching such theory-dense domains. I am encroaching on systems of knowledge that are highly specialised, and in relation to which much theory has been generated. It is not my intention to summarise, explain, or otherwise represent such theory, much less to evaluate it. A significant problem is that the "Western" (European, effectively) perspective on these matters is embedded in an epistemic tradition that is resolutely at odds with traditional perspectives, and the ability to cross from one to the other is fraught with difficulties—in both directions. It is not easy for us to understand the true depth of the relationships that these indigenous people have with "their" plants; and it is not easy for them to understand our atomistic, objectively focused approach. A story that illustrates this goes as follows:

Amazonia is rich territory for scientists seeking new medicinal compounds, and there remains even to this day much yet to be classified and taxonomised in the flora of that area. Typically, many of these "adventure scientists" collaborate with local healers in identifying plants for specific curative uses. The story goes that, having been instructed by local *curanderos* in the medical uses of a particular plant, the scientists took it away and began to experiment with it. After a series of entirely unsuccessful trials, they eventually went back to the local experts and requested further instruction, saying that they had done everything they knew how to do—isolating, assaying, extracting and combining—to make a medicine out of it, but it still didn't "work". The locals considered this, and then asked the question, "Well, did you try talking to the plant?"

One consequence of the nexus with indigenous American spirituality is the appearance of new kid on the herbal block, Plant Spirit Medicine. It was first formulated and brought to the world by Eliot Cowan, who interned with the Huichol Indians in Mexico. Cowan, who was also an acupuncturist, became recognised by that community as an elder, and created a blend of shamanic practices and 5-Elements Chinese medicine theory, which he introduced to the world through his book, *Plant Spirit Medicine: A Journey into the Healing Wisdom of Plants*, first published in 1995.[16] Closely following Cowan are Pam Montgomery[17] (to whom special attention will be given in a later chapter), Sajah Popham,[18] and Davyd Farrell and Emma Fitchett,[19] whose training included time spent with Ecuadorian shaman Kurikindi.[20] It is necessary to understand and to give due credit to the systems and cultures that inspired these examples. They cannot necessarily be bolted onto our local European sensibility without risking significant distortion—although I fully recognise the need to try.

As an educator and writer in the field of what is known as *Western Herbal Medicine* I have learned from experience that "Plant Spirit Medicine" is now an open secret, and many students hunger for it. I am on record as having pronounced that "Western Herbal Medicine is a broad church",[21] but that doesn't mean that all enclaves within that ecumenical community have equal status. To fulfil the requirements of the agreed national core curriculum we must still teach it from a bio-medical, biochemical and *clinical* baseline. We can just about get away with "energetics", as validated by virtue of longstanding and revered global traditions such as Ayurveda and Traditional Chinese Medicine—although the latter is actually a fairly recent aggregate of several different systems reaching back millennia, some of which (arguably in common with all rational systems of medicine), if you look back far enough, have a basis in magic rather than any "rational" system of medicine.[22] But, at all events, we must stick to our "civilised" antecedents.

In Europe, Hippocrates (c.460–c.370 BCE) is referred to as "The Father of Modern Medicine" not because his actual practice, his *materia medica*, or his underpinning philosophical orientation, looked anything like that of modern doctors, but because he, and the body of individuals with whom he worked, and to whose work he gave his name for posterity,[23] were seen in European terms to be proponents of rational, systematic medicine, as distinct from folkloric and "superstitious" practices. His healing practice was in fact largely naturopathic, based on foods, herbs and lifestyle reform.

Contemporaneous with Hippocrates, although arising from quite different cognitive premises, the Cult of Asclepius was based on more ancient and arcane metaphysical principles that predated "rational medicine". Asclepius himself straddles the categories of god and human, and belongs to the heroic era in Greek history, purportedly between 12th and 15th centuries BCE. Asclepius was known to heal people by visiting them in their dreams, and people were still visiting—and spending the night in—his temples, in the expectation of a nocturnal visit, up until 426 CE, when Roman Emperor Theodosius II finally ordered the closure of the Asclepion at Epidaurus following through on the Roman project of Christianisation, and the outlawing of pagan worship.[24]

Interestingly, the practices that replaced the ancient rituals in that location were scarcely more rational than those of Asclepius, as Christian saints took over that function as a matter of course for a few centuries before the site fell into dilapidation, to be rediscovered and excavated by 19th-century archaeologists. However, the process of replacing and overwriting pagan spirituality is a repeating theme of Christian history, most notably—and horrifically—in the witch hunts that took place, mainly in Europe, between 1450 and 1750 CE, in which up to 60,000 people, predominantly women, are thought to have been executed. Less destructively, as we will see in Chapters 8 and 10, was the assimilation by stealth, the best example of which is the calendrical placement of Christmas, the birth of Christ, on the key Pagan festival of Yuletide. This programmatic suppression and assimilation of overtly magical traditions and practices took place in a global context of the establishment of a hegemony of dogmatic, canonical schools of thought, and the attempt to shut down any cognitive system that was seen to operate differently.

Similar "witch hunts" are arguably visible in the history of alternative and complementary medicine, in which the population at large is quite deliberately diverted from healing lineages that predate or challenge the contemporary scientific narratives. Similarly, state-sponsored religion is tolerated as a pacifying gesture, a bribe, to the apparently inerasable fascination with the numinous in the generality of humankind, but to be a "proper" scientist you need to be an atheist, and to be an atheist is to be a wholehearted "rationalist".[25] The net result over centuries of time has been to prise human sensibility apart from any direct apprehension of reality, from personal contact with the spirit world, and from the exercise of frameworks of action and being that arise from such outlying domains of knowledge. Instead, the enforcement of reliance, not to say dependency, on the given narratives, the canons of "science"—or more commonly nowadays, "THE science"—has given rise to the phenomenon of *scientism,* itself commanding quasi-religious authority over the 21st-century human mind.

Scientism, following Robert S. Mendelsohn's critique of medicine,[26] may be described as a "church" in its own right. It has the trappings of an elite ecclesiastical power structure—a bishopric, together with its priesthood, its permitted creed and its cautionary tales. It is the predigestion and necessary simplification of scientific knowledge and its epistemic foundations for delivery to the uninitiated—in rather the same way that the major religions of the world were the public-facing expressions of the ancient mystery traditions. It neatly glosses over the many methodological problems and unresolved complexes of scientific enquiry and presents science as a *fait accompli.* Latterly, it has taken it upon itself to infiltrate social media platforms with grossly oversimplified memes and tropes with which it aims to maintain its hold over the minds of the masses, and to ridicule, vilify and marginalise—not to say cancel and deplatform—anyone who attempts to argue with it or suggest competing ontological perspectives.

The preservation of scientism is especially evident in the management of Wikipedia—formerly an open-access, open-collaboration encyclopaedic internet platform, but which now acts as the self-promoted guardian of "accepted truth". Key areas in scientific enquiry—notably health and medicine—are exclusively reserved to collegiate editing rights and are effectively locked to anyone else who might want to contribute. Entries can be found that refer to alternate or marginalised practices, but these are never represented from within their own structures of knowledge and process. Instead, they are commented upon, as outliers and heretics, and given the tag, "pseudoscience". It is not open to the scientistically uninitiated (or apostatic) to access editing rights to those pages, attempt to set the record straight, or write a defence of such practices.

Thus, culturally dominant themes, and an accepted canon of theoretical knowledge, are presented as *truth,* and few people will argue with them. If you want to complain about the irresponsibility of "climate denial", or "Covid-denial", for example, then you need to point the finger at this hegemonic structure, because what is happening, right now under our noses, is that the foundations of scientific credibility are being undermined by what has replaced true science in the public imagination: a despotic regime that attempts to circumscribe reality within a very narrow range of "hard facts", and a repertory of accepted practices that admits no competition, but which, by the same token, is beginning now to inspire distrust, resistance and apostasy. We are witnessing the stultification of true scientific enquiry (or should we call it basic human curiosity?) and its relegation to a system of mass indoctrination and mind-control. Behind it, well of course, follow the money. KER-CHING.

And so, in a 21st-century higher educational environment feeding into professional practice in a public health context, the tenets of plant spirit medicine are unlikely to form a major strand, for example, in the argument for permissiveness in the face of the drive to regulate traditional medicines, and accordingly we do not teach them in professional herbal training schools. Well, not officially, anyway. There are ways around this, as will become obvious later in this book. Moreover, as we will document in Chapter 6, many of these practices have been heavily colonised by market economies directed at profiting from the sale of commodities derived from the plant world, such that in the public understanding, herbal "supplements" are scarcely distinguishable from any other genre of medicinal or nutritional product.

Summarising, this chapter has attempted to highlight alternate ontologies and the epistemic regimes that flow from them, set against a cultural sensibility that has all but forgotten how to think in any other way than that prescribed by hegemonies of vested interests embedded in state edict, religious injunction and canonical science. The discussion of what, fundamentally, Nature IS, is heavily contaminated by the "official" narratives of the history of science, which itself is generally a recursive editing of historiographic processes. In other words, when it comes to science, ironically, we can and frequently do "make shit up", leaving the question of what, in fact, reality is, entirely open.

* * *

High tide one early September morning at Holkham beach saw marine water edge into the dunes—the first time I have seen this in over 40 years of coming here. I know it can happen—and even in fairly recent history it has occasionally been catastrophic—but I had never seen it with my own eyes. What had appeared yesterday as an expanse of golden sand extending nearly half a mile to the water's edge, is transformed in the bright early morning of today to a placid lake, reaching beyond grass-tufted dunes and sandbanks to the open sea beyond. I know enough about the character of this landscape to expect that when the tide goes out again in a few hours' time, the terrain that I crossed on foot yesterday at low tide, will have changed irrevocably. It seemed a timely metaphor for the ease with which a landscape and a culture, whether physical or virtual, material or psychic, can be overwritten by tides of change and preference, and it caused me to reflect that, in the wider scheme of things, it may be as useless to rail against the tides of political, social or scientific trends as it would be to repeat Canute's experiment and try to hold back the tide here on the North Norfolk coast.

To reach beyond physical restrictions to a locus where our agency becomes a real force is a magical practice. There is nothing flaky, or "woo", about it, and nothing escapist, unrealistic or deluded. To embrace it is not "anti-science". (It may be anti-authority.) It represents a true orientation towards our innermost truth, and the true depth to which this presumed "physical" reality actually reaches once we start to penetrate its secrets. But in pursuit of this project, we need to work collaboratively with our resident co-creators and our spirit helpers, whether human ancestors, totem animals or indeed plants.

On that level, the relegation of plants in human awareness (plant awareness disparity) needs to be reassessed by reference to some of the emerging theory introduced in this chapter. If we take the view (which as we saw earlier is not a true account of evolution even in scientific terms) that there is a hierarchy in creation, and that some life forms are not as important/aware/worthwhile as others, then it is easy to relegate plants by virtue of "lower order" status. But it is a dangerous assumption. It leads to the kinds of misconceptions, omissions, transgressions and exploitations concerning the world at large that I have already alluded to and is part of the mindset that I hope by now readers will agree is not helpful to anyone, including ourselves, in the broad sweep of conditions here on planet earth.

It is time we awoke to the copoietic agency of plants. If we do not, it will not detract one iota from their power base. But it may detract from, and eventually annihilate, our own.

Notes

1. Buhner, S. H. (2004). *The Secret Teachings of Plants: The Intelligence of the Heart in the Direct Perception of Nature.* Rochester, VT: Bear and Company.
2. See https://www.castlewales.com/motte.html for an explanation and some evocative pictures.
3. The term *miasm* is derived from the Greek, *Miasma,* which was originally used by Hippocrates to describe causative mechanisms in disease. Samuel Hahnemann, the founder of Homeopathy, appropriated the concept to refer to the physical and energetic footprints of disease-causing entities that, if not appropriately treated, act as the triggers for

chronic disease processes in the individual, and which may be transmitted as heritable traits to subsequent generations.

4. Attributed to John Anster's translation of a passage in Wolfgang von Goethe's *Faust*.
5. Sender, R., Fuchs, S., Milo, R. (2016). Revised Estimates for the Number of Human and Bacteria Cells in the Body. *PLoS Biology, 14*(8): e1002533. doi: 10.1371/journal.pbio.1002533. PMID: 27541692; PMCID: PMC4991899.
6. Lipton, B. (2015). *The Biology of Belief: Unleashing the Power of Consciousness*. London: Hay House, p. 42.
7. Maturana, H. R. & Varela, F. J. (1980). *Autopoiesis and Cognition: The Realization of the Living*. Dordrecht: D. Reidel.
8. Varela, F. J., Thompson, E., Rosch, E. (1992). *The Embodied Mind: Cognitive Science and Human Experience*. Cambridge, MA: MIT Press.
9. Ibid., p. 9.
10. Di Paolo, E. A., Rohde, M., Hanne De Jaegher, H. (2014). Horizons for the Enactive Mind: Values, Social Interaction, and Play. In *Enaction: Toward a New Paradigm for Cognitive Science*, ed. John Stewar, Oliver Gapenne & Ezequiel A. Di Paolo. Cambridge, MA: MIT Press, pp. 33 ff.
11. Thomas Kuhn and Karl Popper famously debated their respective positions in the same community that gave birth to logical positivism (the Vienna and the Berlin Circles). They are generally perceived to represent opposing positions in the philosophy of science, but on the topic of logical positivism, or logical empiricism, they were united.
12. Kastrup, B. (2019). *The Idea of the World: A Multi-disciplinary Argument for the Mental Nature of Reality*. Iff Books.
13. Goff, P. (2019). *Galileo's Error: Foundations for a New Science of Consciousness*. New York: Pantheon.
14. Mathews, F. (2003). *For Love of Matter: A Contemporary Panpsychism*. Albany, NY: SUNY Press.
15. Roberts, J. (1994). *Seth Speaks: The Eternal Validity of the Soul*. Novato, CA: New World Library.
16. Cowan, E. (2014). *Plant Spirit Medicine: A Journey into the Healing Wisdom of Plants*. Louisville, KY: Sounds True.
17. Montgomery, P. (2008). *Plant Spirit Healing: A Guide to Working with Plant Consciousness*. Rochester, VT: Bear & Company.
18. Popham, S. (2019). *Evolutionary Herbalism: Science, Spirituality, and Medicine from the Heart of Nature*. Berkeley, CA: North Atlantic Books.

19. Farrell, E. (2022). *Journeys with Plant Spirits: Plant Consciousness Healing and Natural Magic Practices*. Rochester, VT: Bear & Company.
20. https://www.kurikindi.co.uk/copy-of-about.
21. Jackson-Main, P. (2005). Western Herbal Medicine—Gender, Culture and Orthodoxy. In: *Reshaping Herbal Medicine: Knowledge, Education and Professional Culture*, ed. Catherine O'Sullivan. London: Elsevier.
22. It has been noted that the practice of moxibustion in Acupuncture may have originated as a magical, ritual practice, echoing the global reputation of the key herb, mugwort, as a bringer of dreams, psychic protection and insight. See Lu, G.-D. & Needham, J. (2002). *Celestial Lancets: A History and Rationale of Acupuncture and Moxa*. Psychology Press.
23. The Hippocratic Corpus is widely thought to have been the work of several authors, not just the one whose memory has survived the processes of historiography.
24. The Theatre of Epidaurus was a major temple sanctified to Asclepius, thought to have been constructed around 340–330 BCE: see https://www.worldhistory.org/timeline/Asclepius/.
25. See Dawkins, R. (2006). *The God Delusion*. London: Bantam.
26. Mendelsohn, R. (1990). *Confessions of a Medical Heretic*. Columbus, OH: McGraw-Hill.

CHAPTER FOUR

The nature of medicine

The art of medicine consists of amusing the patient while nature cures the disease.[1]

I learned to respect and love the Barberry tree, so-called because of the 1-inch thorns (barbs) jutting out from otherwise innocuous-looking branches, and largely invisible when the shrub is in leaf. It was in the garden of Arjuna Wholefoods, a workers' co-operative food retailer on the famous and onetime bohemian Mill Road shopping street in Cambridge. I had been a student at the university in that city, and after a succession of temporary and fairly menial jobs I had landed a position as a co-operative member, which meant that, after a short probation, I was accepted on an equal footing with every other member—no hierarchy, no bosses; a chance to get involved with every aspect of running a natural, organic and vegetarian food supply business with strict ethical principles that aligned almost point for point with my own. It was also ideally suited to my temperament, being (in principle at least) non-hierarchical, and the first step in a long association dealing with plants as commodities as well as medicines—for in addition to foods we also sold a range of dried herbal teas and spices, which were of interest to me as this was shortly after my first encounter with a herbalist as a patient, and I was already captivated.

One day, relaxing in the garden behind the shop with a cup of herbal tea, I stood up to go back in to work, and my head collided with a branch of the tree under which I had sought shelter from the midday sun. Only it was not just the branch, it was one of its barbs, which embedded itself into my scalp so completely that it was impossible to remove it manually—as some of my co-workers tried to do. It was eventually necessary to visit the hospital to have the thing surgically removed.

Strangely, rather than being annoyed, rageful, accusatory or self-pitying, I remember feeling intrigued and amused, and I commented to those around me that it was the sheerest random "accident" that a simple tree had intervened to cause me so much pain and inconvenience. I resolved, once the thorn was excised, to find out about the tree. I found that we were already selling the bark of its root in our herbal section in the shop—barberry bark (*Berberis vulgaris*). It is a remedy for the liver and digestive tract—a liver dredger, bitter tonic, cholagogue, gastrointestinal antiseptic and immunomodulator, its constituent alkaloids reportedly effective against a broad spectrum of bacterial "pathogens", especially in the gut. It is now one of my most frequently used and trusted remedies.

As a toddler, my mother told me, I was an inveterate thumb-sucker. My parents decided to train me out of this habit by smearing my thumb with a proprietary product made from the very bitter gel derived from the aloe plant, which we all called "nasties" (although at my inchoate level of articulacy I apparently referred to it as "shasties"). It was supposed to be a deterrent. I quickly grew to love shasties and at the point when I would start to approach my mother asking for some more, after I had sucked it all off my thumb, she realised that the strategy was not working on me and gave up the effort. Somehow, I obviously stopped sucking my thumb, maybe because after that it lacked the sought-after taste sensation, and so in a way, I guess, the therapy worked.

Bitter aloe is a herbal remedy that I now use in cases of chronic constipation, as also for colon cleansing protocols. It is a powerful anthraquinone-containing laxative, bitter tonic (improves digestive secretions) and anthelmintic (anti-parasitic). Anthraquinones are chemical compounds that have a very bitter taste, and aloe (also known as "bitter aloe") is one of the bitterest of bitters. I apparently established my preference for plant medicine at an early age.

* * *

The term, "heart's desire" is not just an expression, a linguistic usage worn out through over-exposure in the trite narratives of Hollywood movies and romantic novels. It contains the recognition that we are not simply bodies begging for survival, gratefully accepting the crumbs we are thrown by systems too large, too cumbersome for us to influence. As herbalist and author Stephen Harrod Buhner,[2] among many others, reminds us, the heart is an organ of perception. It reaches into the world as our most probing and sensitive channel of knowing, and it signals to us a thousand times a day to let us know if we are on the right track towards fulfilling our most cherished dreams and our most fundamental existential needs. If we are listening.

Recent research has uncovered the astonishing fact that the heart muscle contains taste receptors in its walls that are attuned to the bitter flavour,[3] so it turns out that bitterness is also cardiotonic: who knew? Well, apparently the ancient Chinese did, as we find in the *Huang-di Neijing*, the Yellow Emperor's Classic of Medicine, that the bitter flavour most specifically enters, not the digestion, liver or gall bladder, but the heart.[4] Most cardiac glycosides (powerful heart tonics such as digoxin) have a bitter taste. Once again, we find this constitutional resonance, expressed in molecular language, between the plant world and our human physiology. As my friend and colleague Peter Conway observed, we are naturally "hardwired" to the medicine of plants.[5]

I discussed the heart in Chapter 2, in terms of the principle of exchange—the necessary and self-perpetuating give and take that sustains the natural world. At the end of that chapter I also referred to the notion of "enlightened self-interest", the perception that what benefits you also benefits me. What enriches the community also enriches every individual within it. But in talking of your "heart's desire", I am not necessarily excluding things that you may see as "purely materialistic" and therefore commonly disapproved of or proscribed in pursuit of a "spiritual" or ethical life. Whatever you want—or think you want—a Mercedes-Benz, a yacht, a holiday in the Caribbean, a healthy bank account, (yet another guitar?)—I dare to suggest that these things too may be medicine, at least in the short term. I am not suggesting we accord them more than temporal significance, but if you were to ask me, is it OK to have things that you enjoy, I say absolutely! I certainly do not want your psychological integrity split any further than it already is by proscribing experiences to which you may feel yourself entitled. As long as their acquisition does not hurt anyone else, and as long as you do, in fact, enjoy them. And there, as they say, is the rub.

When it comes to it many have observed that they would happily give up *having things* in exchange for a return to physical health, renewal of a failed relationship, or the return to health (or even the very life) of an important loved one. But the point is, if you cannot enjoy the here and now, whatever it brings, then you are probably going to be unresponsive to any other good that your fancy parades in front of you as necessary or conducive. It will rapidly lose its sparkle as your default mentality reasserts itself—the so-called "suntan" effect—leaving you wanting more, but unable to identify what, in fact, you really do want.

Healing, and meaning, always derive from internally consistent narratives and processes, which are *constitutional*, that is, they are closely aligned to our energy pattern, our intimate personal energetic signature and our purpose in life. In a manner of speaking, no one, however expert, however well-trained, however experienced, can override your self-determination in healing. Of course, we may see professional "healers"—I make a good living out of being one—but the true role of such people is to catalyse, to inspire, to teach, to inform, and thereby to gain consent and generate commitment to the path, and the *experience*, of healing—whatever, in each individual case, that might be.

In contemporary European cultural terms,[6] the term *medicine* has been annexed to a narrow and very specific set of descriptors, largely having to do with the way that medicines are packaged, sold and prescribed, and comprising a socially and industrially recognised and legally sanctioned regime of practices to which entry is forbidden to those who have not earned the requisite credentials. I am not even saying there is anything wrong with this—I am glad that the surgeon performing my appendectomy in 1966 was "properly trained" and knew what he was doing.

But the circumscribing of the function of healing within this narrow and privileged grouping has gone hand in hand with the marginalising of concurrent but ontologically diverse and frequently more ancient practices and is a sociopolitical development that has been at least 300 years in the making. It has culminated in the creation of a global hegemony of colossal proportions, which has succeeded in embedding itself into state political, educational and legislative structures around the world and created an elite class of medicine makers (the pharmaceutical industry) and therapy providers (the medical profession). It is relatively immune from regulation or reform, except along lines decided within its own terms of reference, and it resists all forms of competitive disciplines by a dual, interlinked process of legislative monopoly and methodological categorisation.

The word *medicine*, however, can be found to have very different meanings in other cultural contexts, even today. For example, the "medicine wheels" of the indigenous traditions of America, which are mandalas whose function is to act as a topography of the physical and spiritual orientation of the individual within the natural environment, and which have been shown to have calculable, evidential benefits in health promotion.[7] Or the *medicina* of the Ayahuasqueros of Amazonia, which is far more than the DMT molecule and its enabling harmine alkaloids, and embraces a cosmology of healing that is deeply rooted in ancestral wisdom, the natural world and the spirit realm. More of this later.

In point of fact, literally anything can be a medicine, or a poison, depending on the direction in which it propels you—that is, towards or away from healing—and as we will see, the difference can be difficult to establish. On the salutary side, a chance encounter; a spectacular view; a delicious meal; a personal or professional accolade or award; a domestic animal or pet; a period of convalescence (not a popular prescription these days); a new outfit; a song, poem or painting; watching butterflies on a summer's day; wild swimming; a garden. But in other contexts, all of them may assume quite other characteristics—too much food, the setting of expectations that in time become restrictive, the illness or death of a cherished pet, too much time on your hands, a faulty seam in the outfit, an annoying earworm of a tune, pesky insects that spoil your open-air relaxation, or a garden that refuses to be tamed. Are not these things also, *in an appropriate dose*, medicine, or at least teachers, in their fashion?[8]

We have already assessed the impact of being "in" nature, among green plants (or any other colour come to that) as "clinically" validated in the healing stakes. What I am saying here is that healing is, or can be, many things, but perhaps above all it is an enhanced state of physical, mental and spiritual wellbeing, and anything that induces that state, even by invoking a comparative negative (like cures like?), can be medicine. Eventually, of course, it's up to us. Eventually we may learn to reproduce that state wherever we are, even in circumstances we deem unconducive—some might say that being able to maintain equilibrium and bliss *in spite of* adverse circumstances, including illness, is the truest goal to aim for.

An in-depth study of plant medicine will bring certain principles into clear focus, even on a pharmacological level. The most obvious mistake made by lay people trying to grasp the essence of herbal medicine is to think of herbs as "natural" replacements for drugs. They will point out that pharmaceuticals were originally derived from plants, and give examples such as aspirin from white willow bark, or digoxin from foxglove. While these cases are nominally true (although in both cases there are qualifying factual details to add for the academically meticulous), they do nothing to illustrate the way that herbs actually work.

For example, even on a pharmacological basis, acetylsalicylic acid was originally isolated from the plant *Filipendula ulmaria* (meadowsweet), and only later from *Salix alba* (white willow). Now, of course, like most pharmaceuticals, it's made from petrochemicals—by-products of the oil industry. Meadowsweet even gave aspirin its name: the older Latin name was *Spirea filipendula*, and the name *aspirin* was taken from *Spirea*. Most of us know that a significant side-effect of the long-term use of aspirin is damage to the stomach lining and the triggering of gastroesophageal reflux. That's why people on "gold-standard" pharmaceutical regimes that include aspirin for cardiovascular disease prophylaxis are now routinely prescribed drugs to suppress stomach acid. Now consider that meadowsweet is a herb that we give to people who have gastritis and gastroesophageal reflux disease. So, the herb that contains the all-important anti-inflammatory constituent acetylsalicylic acid, also contains mucilaginous principles that prevent it from harming the stomach. This is an example of nature's protective chemistry, and the reason why the popular notion (not so popular with the pharmaceutical companies) of herbs being "safer" than drugs remains largely true, despite obvious examples where it is not.

For, on that basis we also have herbs that, if not handled correctly, may not be entirely safe. In fact, many herbs (as we just saw) have constituents that can cause harm. The fact that they do not do so is usually a function of their presence in very small, "clinically insignificant" amounts, or in combination in the overall pharmacological profile with compounds that are benign and protective. However, there are herbs whose clinical effectiveness is precisely due to compounds that have the potential to cause actual and lasting harm, and our other example, *Digitalis purpurea* (purple foxglove), is such a herb. Digoxin, a powerful cardiac glycoside isolated from foxglove and used in standard medicine to treat congestive heart failure, has what is called a narrow therapeutic index or margin, which means that it is clinically effective within a very tight dose range. Too little, and it won't do the job. Too much, and it will stop your heart and kill you. This is why the plant is "POM" (prescription only medicine) in UK drug legislation, as it is near impossible to tell exactly how much digoxin an individual plant contains, and therefore to calibrate the dose that should be given. In a pharmaceutical context this is very closely monitored and managed, and the patient will also usually be told about hazards that may accrue to the co-consumption of certain foods and other herbal medicines, which may alter the pharmacokinetics of the drug and therefore either increase or decrease its plasma concentration.

But there is an in-between category: herbs that contain principles that will probably not actually kill you but could cause problems if consumed in unwise amounts. In this regard we need first to reflect that current accepted theory, in terms of the derivation of what are called "secondary plant metabolites", many of which are at the forefront of the pharmacological explanations of how herbs "work", is still resolutely pharmacological, and therefore essentially reductionist in focus. These substances, it is thought, are developed in plants as means of defence against predators, or sometimes as an attraction to pollinators or species that could provide benefit by interacting with the plant. Even if you want to look at things in purely chemical terms, however, there begins to emerge a wider field of possibilities, and this is part of the biochemical apparatus that drives the phenomena I discussed in Chapter 2. In that discussion I hypothesised, along with other key commentators, that plants are here to give us their goods in exchange for something, and that that exchange is not necessarily something we have to "agree to", explicitly, but is actually integral to the conditions of life on earth—so much so that we do not even see it happening, unless we are researching the matter a little deeper, as we are here.

Taking it further, we might also observe that in traditional healing using plants, the experience is not always pleasant. In other words, the "chemicals" in the plants, aside from occasionally being responsible for an "unpleasant" taste (a highly subjective evaluation, as we saw from my aloe consumption experiment in childhood), can also act, for example, as purgatives, emetics, diaphoretics, stimulants and narcotics. Anyone who has partaken of *la medicina* in an Amazonian context will be very familiar with the sometimes-terrifying onset of profound nausea and violent purging in the early stages of ingestion. This is part of how the medicine accomplishes its effects, and participants will often report that along with the physical purging there is also an emotional purging that takes place at this stage of the ceremony. The idea is that we need to offload the sickness-promoting material as effluent, before we are ready to receive the gift of enhanced insight and bliss that the medicine is also able to provide.

But this is an extreme category, and not one that many patients of herbalists seek out—for understandable reasons. Purgation, diaphoresis and emesis appear as functions of a number of commonly used herbs in professional practice, and even in over-the-counter medications. Senokot, for example, a brand name for a product containing anthraquinone glycosides extracted from the plant *Cassia angustifolia*, or senna, is a well-known remedy for constipation. If I took this product, I don't mind telling you that it would promote a purge with symptoms that, if consulting a doctor, would probably be diagnosed as irritable bowel syndrome—in other words it would make me feel "unwell". Obviously for others that does not happen (or it wouldn't be licensed for general sale), but the fact that I personally do not need it does not render it a poison, and I use the plant in my own practice, judiciously and alongside other plants (notably aloe) for the treatment of constipation, and as part of a colon cleansing protocol.

Purgation and emesis, however, along with bloodletting, were and are permissible actions for use in traditional medicine categories, no matter that the typical patients of the contemporary era have been softened too far to accept them. The renowned American Eclectic herbalist, Dr John Christopher, for example, used the plant *Lobelia inflata* very frequently for its superior antispasmodic action, but also in a well-known specific protocol to treat asthma attacks. At a certain dose (which may be different for each person, requiring careful titration) the ingested plant triggers the gagging reflex at the back of the throat, causing vomiting. As a one-time chronic asthma sufferer, I can report knowledgeably on the effectiveness of the treatment, and I have also used it on suitably informed and consenting subjects in my professional practice. Lobelia contains the alkaloid *lobeline*, which is chemically similar to nicotine—the other major use for lobelia is as a substitution protocol for people who want to stop smoking (you can imagine how carefully this needs to be done). In the UK lobelia is a Schedule 20 herb, which means that it is permitted for exclusive use by appropriately trained professional practitioners and comes with statutory maximum single and weekly doses.

I once attended an Amazonian tobacco ceremony based upon the consumption of tobacco tea. It was not pleasant, but I was intrigued to note that it resulted in the same scratchy feeling in the back of my throat coupled with nausea, very similar to that I had experienced from the asthma treatment using lobelia. Another Amazonian healing practice uses powdered tobacco, sometimes mixed with other psychoactive herbs. Rapé (or hapé) is blown forcibly up the nostril through a special pipe designed for the purpose, resulting in a blinding flash of what I can only describe as intense pain, before triggering nausea in a very similar way. In the interests of balanced reporting, I would have to add that once you get used to it, the experience can be exhilarating and instructive and has the power to clear out both physical and energetic blockages very quickly. The point I am reinforcing is that there is sometimes a fine line between a poison and a cure. We will discuss tobacco again as we reach further into the subject matter of this book.

The use of strong purgative herbs, the use of UK listed Schedule 20 herbs, the use of *heroic* herbs, is not the daily bread of a herbalist. Most of the time we are engaged in far more gentle regimes of cleansing, balancing, harmonising, promoting, releasing and perhaps even inspiring through mood enhancement. But we also admit that the less comfortable experiences can nonetheless be salutary in the wider scheme of things, and perhaps even necessary. This basic principle can also include "negative" life events: there is a tendency to emphasise the traumatising effects of such events, but as I discussed in a previous book,[9] they can also serve to awaken, reset, clarify, restructure and detoxify—in the sense of clearing out what no longer serves. Pain and discomfort are often a part of the healing, and of the teaching.

Even where they are not, however, there are clarifications to be made in circumscribing the scope of any remedy. A true understanding of herbal medicine reveals that the focus is far more frequently on the pathogenesis, or the pathophysiology, rather than the pathology as a discrete entity. In other words, practitioners are more interested in determining how the condition comes about than in defining and naming the "condition" itself. For example, in a case of constipation, we can take a "heroic" herb such as aloe or senna, which will effectively force a result by triggering a contraction of peristaltic muscles. In some cases, where for example the causation is excessive tension in these muscles, this will be exactly the wrong thing to do and may cause griping and spasm or even intense pain. Clearly, we need to investigate the underlying reason for the retentive condition. Occasionally it may indeed be diagnosed as weakness or flaccidity of the musculature, but far more frequently it will be found in conditions higher up the causal chain. These might be manifesting as a shortfall of digestive secretions, particularly bile from the liver, which is a natural laxative. The appropriate response here is to use herbs that stimulate the production and secretion of bile—choleretics and cholagogues.

There might also be psychosomatic factors in play: how many of us have experienced either constipation or indeed diarrhoea as a response to stressful physical or emotional events? In such a case there would be a need perhaps for relaxants and anxiolytics. At the simplest, constipation may signal dehydration—the colon absorbs water from the faecal matter passing through. If it is already dried out, this will dry it further and impede its elimination. The remedy? Water! And perhaps the action of lubricating, mucilaginous herbs such as marshmallow root or slippery elm bark powder—although be aware that these also will absorb a significant amount of water.

The category of *Alterative* herbs is another example. In fact, many plants have "alterative" properties, no matter that they may also have other actions and principles. The word—an old medical term—means to gradually alter a pathological state by addressing a complex range of potential causative factors, by various means of clearing and detoxifying, nourishing and strengthening, relaxing or toning, and by modulating immune, circulatory, digestive and neurological parameters. The alterative is found among the most abundant herbal actions out there in the plant world, and I can think of few cases indeed where the right alterative would not be appropriate. Their indications (conditions for which they are prescribed) include headache and migraine, constipation, digestive deficiency, parasitic infestation, liver congestion, water retention, skin problems, immune deficiency, respiratory distress, rheumatic and arthritic disease (including autoimmune presentations), circulatory disease (especially ischaemic—blocking of arterial vessels), chronic and post-viral fatigue, infertility, depression and anxiety, diabetes and cancer. Among many other possibilities.

A key word in describing the effects of the alterative herbs is "gradually". They are not generally heroic herbs—although some herbs that can be used heroically, such as cayenne and garlic, are also classified as alteratives. They are more often gentle cleansers, restoratives and nutritives, and are therefore widely tolerated, and have very broad applications. They do not, however, suppress symptoms to provide instant relief, and so at a certain point their use—and the category itself—was discontinued in mainstream medicine and left to the plant healers.

There's a need to flag up a misconception around the word "allopathic". It has been synonymised with standard, mainstream medicine, which is indeed largely allopathic in nature, but it is more than its association with any one medical practice or tradition. The prefix *allo-* means 'other', and stands in contrast to *homeo-*, which means 'the same'. Homeopathy, therefore, treats like with like. Allopathic approaches, treating with opposites, as judicious responses to certain symptomatic phenomena, are justified and useful in some circumstances. Extreme and painful episodes of tension and contraction call for release, so that the flow of vital energy can be restored and might require the use of an *anti*-spasmodic. In Chinese medicine the phenomenon of "perverse heat" caused by stagnation can be addressed with "heat-clearing" herbs, which are most often cool, or cold, in quality, and which relieve and disperse the build-up. Although inflammation is a physiological healing mechanism, and must not be summarily suppressed and erased, if rampant and unregulated it may frequently be painful and destructive, and therefore undesirable, calling for *anti*-inflammatory action. In cases where the system is unable to regulate itself, allopathic approaches may be deployed, judiciously, in the effort to restore homeostasis and preserve life. In that way the inherent, indwelling vital energy, and therefore the healing, may best be preserved and enabled. And although in Chapter 6 I am going to subject the *anti-* prefix to some critical comment, it is important for balance to include this perspective.

These explanations are intended to flesh out what practitioners of plant medicine actually do, and the particular view they may take of "disease" processes and their causes; and thereby how to select the appropriate therapeutic responses, including but not limited to the choice of plant medicines. It is a highly complex matter, as humans are complex beings, and we prize medicinal plants for their ability to match that complexity in the range of actions and modulations that they can perform. Natural medicine interventions also tend to be complex outside of the choice of plant remedies, and this is where we recognise that literally anything has the potential to be "medicine". In all areas of our lives where we have choice and agency there is the possibility to move towards either health, which is wholeness and harmony, or towards illness, which is compartmentalisation and incoherency.

Further, it is an established principle of natural health practice that we teach the methods of self-regulation in healthcare, and desist from coercion and mandate in favour of persuasion and example. It is my own point of view that it might be necessary on occasion to recognise that the person may need to move deeper into his or her distress through "doing the wrong things" until they discover for themselves that these things have served their purpose. It's a fine judgment call, but in such cases, prohibition and dogmatic precept rarely work.

Plants, herbs and spices especially, once possessed rare value in terms of commodities and trade. They still do, to a far lesser extent, but have been largely displaced in the contemporary market by the proprietary products of the pharmaceutical and chemical industries. You cannot patent a naturally occurring plant—a fact that has drawn howls of protest from those industries when they realised that herbal products in "their" market were subject to very little regulatory oversight and therefore represented unfair competition. When you spend millions on the research, development and licensing of pharmaceuticals, the idea that someone can dig up a root and apply it as an effective medicine is an irksome and unwanted feature of the commercial landscape, as is the idea that people might have easy access to healing materials and principles that sidestep the profit-motive of these monopolising cartels. This single factor has been responsible for multiple attempts to "regulate" plant medicine out of existence—with greater or lesser levels of success depending on the inherent legislative permissiveness of individual nation states. Plant medicine, in its purest form, quite naturally resists recruitment to monopolising and hegemonic agendas, and that fact was pivotal in the epiphany that I described in my own life at the beginning of Chapter 3.

We are coming closer, in this thesis, to the point at which we will need to approach the true nature of plants themselves. We may well find that their true nature is, in fact, closer to our own than we may have imagined. But we are not usually aware of this possibility, and our general state tends to be one of relative darkness. Even where we may happen upon crumbs of enlightenment that temporarily illuminate our worlds, there is usually a quick return to the usual mindset and a capitulation to received and accepted values, and perceptions that serve mundane purposes and keep the *status quo* intact—business as usual. In this we will find, once we know how to access it, the ageless wisdom of the plants themselves can assist us to stay focused on the antidote. Not just the superstars—the heroics, the entheogens and the so-called "master plants"—but even the smallest and most humble of plants. Once you know how to regard them.

* * *

A vivid electrical flash interrupts my train of thought, followed a few seconds later by a ricocheting peal of thunder and a ferocious, barely announced deluge. The field of vision in front of me is blurred with the cascading water, even though I can already see edges of pewter light above the distant trees, signalling the imminent passing of the storm. I am reminded of hexagram number 51 of the *I-Ching, the Book of Changes*: Thunder. In fact, the hexagram is composed of a doubling of the trigram of thunder, a repeating pattern, top three and bottom three:

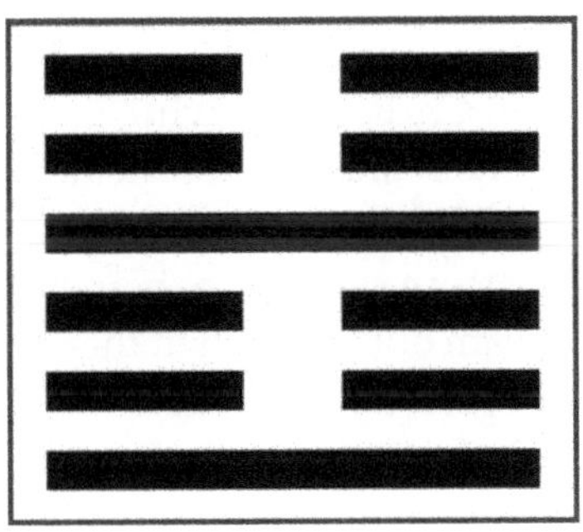

I have always loved thunder. It arouses excitement and the promise of possibilities beyond rational thought. From the Wilhelm/Baynes translation, the following meaning is derived:

> *Shock brings success. Shock comes—oh, oh! Laughing words—ha, ha! The shock terrifies for a hundred miles, and he does not let fall the sacrificial spoon and chalice.*[10]

Thunder initiates action through shaking the foundations of thought—action that stimulates and perpetuates movement along the chosen path. The action that generates a thousand actions. As the early evening sun reestablishes itself, the warm rays penetrating through the rain-spotted window, I reflect that this could work as a metaphor for a healing event. The shock of the symptom, the pain, or the diagnosis as internal communication, giving way to the reassurance that in sticking to one's principles (the establishment of healing protocol) success is assured, and thus redoubling efforts to follow through. A wake-up call, maybe. Thunder has always been an important medicine for me.

Similarly, plants that have attracted the epithet "heroic" in medicinal use may be regarded in a similar light, and have always resonated. Plants of the Solonaceae (nightshade) family, in particular, tend to have this property. The most famous of these in standard herbal use is capsicum (cayenne pepper). Most often thought of as a food-flavouring spice (with the specific contribution of extraordinary "heat"), the addition of capsicum to a personalised herbal formula is rarely welcomed by the average patient, however it can be extremely salutory. I have been berated more times than I could mention for the practice of adding a very small amount of capsicum to an eyewash formula. In fact it was not my idea—it was a formula I learned from my herbal professor, Dr Schulze, who himself acquired it from the late great American Eclectic herbalist, Dr John Christopher, who himself may have received it from his association with indigenous healers from the American Indian populations, for certain tribal healers and shamans are known to place crushed hot capsicum seeds into their eyes to enhance spiritual sight. Many patients scream out loud when they first apply this remedy, and many of them then pick up the phone and scream some more at me. As noted above, pain is often a part of the healing. But wait a few moments for the sting to subside, and there is a euphoric sensation of clarity and light, emanating specifically from enhanced vision and the clearing away of obfuscations and fearfulness.

Shock! Oh, oh! Then laughter, ha ha!!

Notes

1. This satirical quip is attributed to French philosopher and writer François-Marie Arouet, AKA Voltaire, but sources are obscure, with some suggesting that the quote, or a version of it, was in circulation before Voltaire was born, possibly originating with Jean-Baptiste Poquelin, AKA Molière, the French playwright.

2. Buhner, S. H. (2004). *The Secret Teachings of Plants: The Intelligence of the Heart in the Direct Perception of Nature*. Rochester, VT: Bear and Company.
3. Bloxham, C. J., Foster, S. R., Thomas, W. G. (2020). A Bitter Taste in Your Heart. *Frontiers in Physiology,* 11: 431. doi: 10.3389/fphys.2020.00431. PMID: 32457649; PMCID: PMC7225360.
4. Ni, M. (1995). *The Yellow Emperor's Classic of Medicine*. Boulder, CO: Shambhala.
5. Conway, P. (2010). *The Consultation in Phytotherapy*. London: Elsevier.
6. My use of the term *European* relates to a cultural orientation, not a demographic or geopolitical entity. The dominant civilisations of the Americas, and of the antipodes, Australia and New Zealand, are essentially European in character. It is the case that this orientation is difficult indeed to avoid today, wherever in the world you travel. In terms of economic priorities, medical responses, legal processes, with few exceptions the term *civilised* is a largely synonym for *Europeanised.*
7. Dapice, A. N. (2006). The Medicine Wheel. *Journal of Transcultural Nursing, 17*(3): 251–260.
8. Hormesis is the scientific elaboration of the notion that "what does not kill makes me stronger", originally attributed to the German philosopher Friedrich Nietzsche. It is the way in which adversity and challenge, physiological or psychological, helps us to develop resilience, strength and skill.
9. Jackson-Main, P. (2025). *Natural Healing: Staying Well Naturally in the Modern World*. London: Aeon.
10. *I Ching, or Book of Changes*. (1989). Richard Wilhelm translation. London: Arkana/Penguin.

CHAPTER FIVE

Plants or products: the decolonisation of herbal practice

Asking what distinguishes us from the others—and it makes little difference who "they" are, since really what matters in that case is only "us"—is already a response.

Eduardo Viveiros de Castro[1]

I was filming a "herb walk" on a large private estate in East Sussex. The idea of a herb walk is that the "expert" herbalist guides and directs his audience in discovery and discussion of the flora encountered on the walk. Usually, he or she will have first scouted the territory and prepared the itinerary, knowing which plants will present themselves along the way. Because we were filming for online educational content, and both time and budget had to be managed carefully, on this occasion I went "sight unseen", trusting and expecting that what we needed to see would appear.

The estate consisted largely of managed agricultural land, mainly a collection of rolling meadows and fields, framed and interspersed with woods that burgeoned with bluebell, primrose and wild garlic in season, and streams that offered habitat to mallow, horsetail and butterbur. Woods were bordered and protected by banks of nettle, as were the solitary oaks that stood majestically in one or two of the fields. In the woods and along the verges of the woodland tracks we encountered variously elder, hawthorn, dog rose, oak, horse chestnut, hazel, lime and various birch species, while the extensive meadows hosted ribwort plantain, yarrow, fennel and various species of dock (*Rumex*), and there was one field of cultivated red clover—*Trifolium pratense*, "three-leaved of the meadow"—a cover crop destined to be ploughed back into the land for the purpose of nitrogen-fixing for the benefit of future cash crop plantings.

I have mentioned mainly the commonly recognised medicinal plants, but there were many other unsung species and modest heroes, and an occasional moderate rarity, such as an encounter with *Angelica sylvestris*, a member of the genus that also gives us the northern European species *A. archangelica* (digestive and circulatory stimulant) and the exotic Asian *A. sinensis* (Dong Quai, blood nourisher and blood mover, female hormonal modulator), and of the family *Apiaceae*, which gives us fennel, celery, carrot and parsley, among many other useful and delicious food plants. There was no shortage of plants to engage with and expound upon, and in fact we ended up returning seasonally throughout the year of the pandemic, when there were few indeed of our own kind to bother us as we rambled to our hearts' content, two cameramen and one happy herbalist, all appropriately socially distanced, of course.

The moment of peak aesthesis came when, upon pushing open a creaking, tarnished alloy gate, I was quite suddenly confronted with a spectacular vista of dandelion in full bloom across an undulating green landscape of maybe 5 or 6 acres. Thousands, tens of thousands of bright yellow heads poking up through the unmown grass of the meadow, a carpet of golden suns waving gloriously at me and inviting me to step among them and immerse myself in their pure golden joy.

What we call "dandelion" represents around 250 species, in the UK and Ireland alone, within the genus *Taraxacum*. *Taraxacum* comes from the Arabic *tarakhshaqun*, meaning "bitter herb".[2] Even if you are not a herbalist and have read thus far in this book you might already have worked out what one or two of its medicinal benefits might be. The medicinal species is designated by the Latin *Taraxacum officinalis*, but there are many, many other species and sub-species and some of them are almost impossible to tell apart—even experienced botanists can argue over them for hours. In herbal medicine the question is often asked, does it matter what species? Sometimes yes, sometimes no. In terms of dandelion, since the chances of misidentification are so high,

I'd warrant that much of the material that reaches the herbalist's shelf is not *officinalis*, but one of the alternate or sub-species. It doesn't seem to matter. At the end of the day, as they say, suck it and see.

Organolepsy, the practice of deploying your own five senses to deliver information about medicinal plants, will tell you that the plant is indeed bitter—the leaf especially, although the root also has a content of sweet principles—immunomodulatory complex sugars alongside the "warm bitter" principles of the sesquiterpene lactones. The herb is celebrated as one of the most broadly applicable and widely tolerated alteratives in the *materia medica*, acting on both liver and kidneys to promote the self-cleansing, as well as the self-nourishing processes of the body.

But it was the heart-promoting benefits that immediately recommended themselves to me on that bright, early summer day in Sussex. Not usually referred to as a heart tonic of any description, dandelion is in my view one of the most uplifting herbs—certainly visually, but also medicinally, since it is one of the most effective liver dredgers in the *materia medica*. Liver dredging can chase out a whole catalogue of ills resulting from toxic, stagnant substance and energy, as well as emotion—particularly resentment, entrenched anger and grudge-bearing, blame, frustration and depression. If the liver is stressed, overburdened and stagnant, we reflect those qualities in our mood.

Dandelion is also the herb featured in a well-known TV advert for the chemical product *Roundup*, which is a glyphosate-containing weed-killer. Watching the advert, we are supposed to take deep satisfaction in the sight of a member of the dandelion family wilting, shrivelling and dying in fast-motion after an application of the magic potion. Because we all hate dandelions, don't we? Nasty, invasive things that spoil our lawns and can't be dug out owing to a tap root that can penetrate up to eight feet into the earth. You can try, but what will happen is that the root will snap, and what is left in the ground will very quickly supply another perfect plant. So, let's "treat" the "problem" with a noxious poison (one that also poisons us owing to its widespread use in agriculture), that penetrates via the leaves, down the stems, and into the remotest parts of the root structure. Job done. Back to the sun lounger.

Except that, fortunately, trying to get rid of dandelions is like trying to get rid of unsolicited phone calls from people selling PPI insurance: no matter how many times to you tell them that you have exhausted your PPI compensation entitlement and you don't need their service, there's always another one, and another, and another. "Good morning Peter, how are you today?" (From dandelion that would be a worthy greeting!) In the case of dandelion, however, the supreme irony is that this is a plant that can detoxify us from the worst excesses of our own ingenuity. It can quite easily overcome and destroy its own nemesis. It may even be that dandelion uses the information delivered in the poisoning to make it more effective as a solution to that poisoning. Scientifically we might refer to that as "developing tolerance", in the same way that bacteria learn how to resist and survive antibiotics. But by extension, hypothetically speaking, they may also be performing a global, not merely a selfish, purpose, as do many plants, in absorbing, breaking down and neutralising toxic residues, both in the environment and in our own bodies, and thus potentially serve as an antidote to the widespread problem of human poisoning through glyphosate and other noxious inventions of the chemical industries.

My good friend and spiritual brother, plant shaman Davyd Farrell, once said of dandelion (*El Dandelero*, as he affectionately calls him), *"This guy is a master geneticist and a time lord. He can create hundreds of thousands of versions of himself simultaneously around the whole world and throughout time and history. I can't do that!"* That's a very good point. What kind of organising principle, what kind of energy essence, what kind of *being*, is able to perform this trick? It doesn't apply to dandelions alone of course: all plants, to one extent or another, can do this, or something close to it. Some maintain a strictly local presence; others, like *El Dandelero*, are the global superstars of the plant world. Dandelion is a cosmic being, poetically described in the observation that the flower symbolises the sun, the silver globe seedhead the moon, and the dozens of anemochoric (wind-dispersed) seeds the stars.

* * *

In the present discussion, the word *decolonisation* is intended to refer to the task of "identifying colonial systems, structures and relationships, and working to challenge those systems".[3] Fundamentally, it is a rethinking of power relations between participants in any transaction. In the case of herbal medicine, this means challenging the commercial exploitation of plants through redefining our relationship with them along democratic and *convivial* lines. In other words, while we view plants as mere commodities, we risk denying them self-definition and agency. But we also simultaneously restrict our own access to the inherent creativity accruing to a more flexible and collaborative approach.

Guy Waddell refers to the ethos of Western Herbal Medicine as an "enchantment".[4] Noting that the architecture of rational systems of medicine, even in revered traditional modalities such as TCM and Ayurveda, is constituted by the paraphernalia of linguistic usages and foundational concepts—such as *qi*, *prana*, *yin* and *yang*, the elements, the *doshas* and temperaments, the various tissue states, and so forth—he proposes that the constitutional signifiers of Western Herbal Medicine, in place of these lexical forms, are Nettle, Dandelion, Yarrow, Hawthorn, and so on. In other words, he suggests, it is the plants themselves that define our practice.

Western Herbal Medicine could indeed be framed as a system-less system: one that has lost its epistemic roots in terms of an underlying rationale (although perhaps for that all the more redolent with folkloric and intuitive usages) while also, paradoxically, mirroring a concept of "specific" medicine that we might naturally—if naively—associate with standard pharmaceutical medicine. A herb for every ailment: a pill for every ill.

This apparent simplicity, however, may lead to a misinterpretation of Western Herbal Medicine, in three key respects. Firstly, it may cause us to regard plant medicines as being similar to pharmaceutical medicines, but "natural". Secondly, the plants themselves become imprisoned in a template, or grid, of human usage, meaning that people tend to *think* of plants in the same way they think of drugs, and therefore to interact with them in the same way. Plants then become secondary to the systematic practice—incidental, given meaning and purpose only in relation to the epistemological preferences of the canon of medicine, rather than being central to it, let alone having agency in their own right. And thirdly, practitioners of Western Herbal Medicine are too often assumed to be ersatz versions of "real" doctors—which is a two-edged sword, as for some this will be a selling point, for others a condemnation. A fourth distortion, which is the central theme of this chapter, is that all of this enables a commercial environment in which plants are mere commodities: there for the realisation of profit as the primary motivation of those who trade in them.

Many practitioners of Western Herbal Medicine were profoundly influenced by the influx, during the 1960s, of Chinese doctors setting up practice in the UK. They saw in TCM, and later in Ayurveda, something that we didn't have (or perhaps had forgotten) in European medicine. So fascinated were they, and so critical of their own tradition, that many freely admitted that they jumped ship on to these venerable—but culturally distant—versions of herbal and natural medicine. Even the Physiomedicalist schools, hailing from North America and imported into the UK by the unfortunately named Albert Isaac Coffin in 1838, were not considered sufficiently robust for the new generation of UK herbalists, who, hypnotised by the prevailing scientific ethos, became polarised into *phytotherapists*, holding a resolutely objectivist scientific ethic, or advocates of exotic offshore systems such as TCM and Ayurveda. A few retreated into "hedgerow herbalism"—a return to feudal foraging and folkloric fellowship—no bad thing, indeed.

I was talking among colleagues about this at professional event a couple of decades ago. Bemoaning the fact that Galenic humoral theory had not survived the enlightenment, we turned over the possibility of reigniting that tradition. It never really happened. Both TCM and Ayurveda are living traditions, with a continuity stretching over millennia. The Galenic humoral tradition was violently disrupted and displaced at a certain era in European culture. I did work it into the curriculum of the course I administer but had to admit it was far from a complete, workable system, although to be fair, David Osborn's *Greek Medicine* website is a heroic attempt to reinsert this venerable tradition into a contemporary dialogue.[5] Middle Eastern medicine, or *Unani Tibb*, is the closest surviving tradition, and has clung on by a thread in the UK, thanks to a couple of small but active schools, and a recent welcome addition to natural healing literature courtesy of my colleague, Shahid Burkhari.[6]

Waddell's thesis, then, was a welcome championing of a little-suspected strength, and if I am honest, and despite the highly developed artisanry in medicine- and formula-making typical of our more ancient traditional cousins, I did not, and still do not, see the deeper medicine that accrues uniquely to the plant world, which I am trying to foreground in this book, reflected in these systems. In general terms they might be talking about anything: rocks, dust, insects, pottery, rainwater… In both Chinese and Ayurvedic medicine indeed, animal and mineral substances do indeed appear in the *materia medica* alongside plants (begging very similar questions in relation to those entities). The point for this thesis is, what tribute is paid to *plants* in any of these systems? Their qualities, in medicinal terms, are well-articulated and praised, but their reality as ontologically distinct agents, undefined by human usage, is notoriously absent from these accounts.

Waddell further proposes, as I discussed in Chapter 2, that plants and humans may function as each other's "convivial tools". In other words, we use each other, but *nicely*, and reciprocally. The word *convivial* implies an easy and familiar co-existence—even a celebratory collaboration. I guess it's similar to Sheldrake's concept of the gifting to humanity of alcohol by fungi? Here at least, the plants can live and breathe as themselves. To what extent, however, are we able to embed that into a *practice* of herbal medicine? To what extent does it permit us to get away from the world of *products*, and bring our clients face to face with their healing allies?

In the early days of our herbal medicine practice, we rented an allotment just at the back of our garden in Cambridge, upon which grew a cornucopia of medicinal plants, some wild, some naturalised through seeding from adjacent plots: nettle, dandelion, dock, comfrey, fennel, yarrow, field poppy, to name but a few. We were usually in trouble with our neighbours on the allotment site, as well as the allotment administrators, who berated us for not "cultivating" our patch, as it was visibly full of "weeds". Our reply, that what was growing there was in fact what we wanted to grow, was met with predictable incomprehension—if not derision. But one plan we had for the land was that we might make it work as a resource for our clients, many of whom pleaded poverty in the face of the charges we made for the "properly produced" medicines that came in bottles or capsules. We began to offer exchanges: come and work on the allotment, gather your own herbal medicines, rather than pay our dispensary prices.

I was in fact replicating an historical precedent. From 1998 to 2011 I worked in a herbal practice in Lancashire known as Abbotts of Leigh. Charles Abbott, the founding practitioner, a physiomedicalist, would do likewise, organising foraging parties on local land to gather the plants he needed for his dispensary. The events, by all accounts (and I did indeed hear several first-hand accounts of these forays), were well-attended, and something of a community occasion. For my own efforts: well, if I report that the number of people who took us up on this offer was precisely ZERO, I think at this stage my readers will probably not be surprised. Was I simply not as charismatic as Charles Abbott? Or have times changed in that regard in the intervening decades? Abbott himself continued to make most of his medicines on the premises—and 15 years after his death, when I joined, the practice manager and her husband, Jean and Peter Berry, were still making them, and continued to do so for the thirteen years of my tenure as the herbalist in Abbotts of Leigh. But even Abbott moved towards proprietary pills and potions for his patent formulae, and indeed outsourced their manufacture, as his reputation grew wider and he found himself not just locally or nationally celebrated, but globally renowned.

The fact is that, poor or not, my own patients were distinctly underwhelmed by the prospect of earning their medicines through hard graft on the land and preferred to buy the products in stock. I suspect that this was only partly laziness (and the fortuitous discovery that they were not, in fact, as poor as they thought they were) but also an endemic distrust of the "ordinary" in favour of the "proper". Somehow, they could trust things that had appropriate labelling (even if it was done on our own dispensary Hewlett-Packard printer on Avery label stock) and came with tamper-evident fastenings. Whereas stuff growing randomly was just weeds, wasn't it? I wonder whether they ever asked themselves what the contents of their bottles and pills had looked like before they were harvested.

Since that time, I have noticed that herbal remedies have increasingly attracted the tag, "supplement" or "product", and I have even used those terms to describe to post office officials what is in the suspicious-looking packages that I send several times a week to our clients. "Supplements" is waived on, unconcerned. "Herbal medicines" immediately prompts further questioning. It reminds me that when we had a high street shop—The Herb Shop—we had occasional visits from plain-clothes officers posing as customers asking if we sold "herb" (the obvious connotation being cannabis). It was the constabulary-issue footwear that gave them away, so we dutifully told them that that would be illegal, whereas what we sold was, in fact, legal, under section 12.2 of the 1968 Medicines Act.[7]

Dr Schulze, our herbal professor, had once shared the opinion that a herbalist should not be able to cross an international border without being intercepted at customs. This was after he himself had been relieved of all his herbal teaching materials by the Spanish border police on his way in to take my first ever Master Class in herbal medicine. The implication was also, that if you choose plant medicine as your go-to health option, you should never be without a basic supply, wherever you go. After all, do not everyday tourists pack paracetamol, ibuprofen, antihistamines, sun cream, Imodium, Rennie, antimalaria pills—in addition to their prescribed medicines—before they board?

In my previous book, *Natural Healing*, commenting on the word *natural* as a marketing tag, I noted that it is common even for students of natural medicine to ask questions such as "What brand should I buy?", on being advised to use a particular herb. What "brand", indeed, is Nature? Out the door, turn left or right, keep walking till you come to a field. Oh… sorry, you've already got some in your garden.

Schulze, again, produced one of the most hilarious teaching videos I ever saw, which saw him standing at a table with a pile of proprietary herbal products in front of him, examining the packaging before ripping it open, smelling and tasting its contents, then consigning it unceremoniously to a large garbage can just next to him. He later told me that he had a lawyer present off-camera, retained for purposes of advice in case he said anything that could get him sued by the mighty quasi-pharmaceutical supplement companies whose wares he was systematically panning. The problem for these companies was that, at the time, not only was the Herb Doc highly influential (that was before the FDA gagged him and tried to remove him from public awareness—too late, as it turned out) but he was also becoming seriously wealthy through the success of his own *American Botanical Pharmacy* and its traditionally produced wares.

When he repeated the trick in a public lecture in Central London in 2013, he shredded a very well-known "immune boosting" tea and scattered the contents over the front two rows of the audience, to universal uproarious laughter, and commented, "FIVE PERCENT Echinacea root in an infusion?? How in hell is that supposed to do anything?" I told him afterwards that the owner of the very well-known herbal tea company was an acquaintance of mine (in fact Anji and I used to work for him) and that he was known for being, let's say, somewhat trigger happy with litigation. Schulze thought for a second or two, mildly concerned, and then observed laconically, "Pretty sure I pay my lawyers more than he does."

In a footnote in *Natural Healing* I also revealed that several major manufacturers of supplements, herbal and/or nutritional (nutraceutical), are now owned by pharmaceutical companies. Why not? Big Pharma cares nothing for epistemological or paradigmatic debates around medicine. It is there for one purpose, and one purpose only: to make money. "If people are buying this stuff, we better be making it. Medicine is *our* patch. These hobos are trespassing."

I was teaching in Temple Bar, Dublin, in 2001, around the time that St John's wort was getting itself into trouble with the regulatory authorities in Europe generally, but in the UK and Ireland specifically. Someone had published an article in *The Lancet*, the journal of the British Medical Association, to the effect that a standardised extract of the plant was as effective for mild to moderate depression as the pharmaceutical market leader (at the time), Prozac. Reportedly, Eli Lilly, the manufacturer of Prozac, lost several billion dollars in revenue directly from this gratuitous publicity.[8] The predictable result was a legislative crackdown on the plant throughout Europe, and it was banned in many countries, including Ireland (but interestingly not the UK), on a pretext of dangerous side effects and contraindications. For example, it was found to induce certain CYP450 liver enzyme detoxification pathways, and thus potentially interfere with a wide range of pharmaceutical drugs, resulting in harm to patients taking these drugs, who might thereby find themselves with lower than desirable plasma concentrations of the active principles. A prime example put forward was the OCP (oral contraceptive pill), whose effectiveness was theoretically reduced by 2 or 3 percentage points in women who were co-administering St John's wort alongside their contraception. This had purportedly so far resulted in a statistic of 14 unwanted pregnancies, and as one colleague joining the call for caution in prescribing St John's wort tautologously put it, "No one wants an unwanted pregnancy."

What was not said, which remains to this day the elephant in the room, was that the plant constituents found to be responsible for these effects were none other than the flavonoids—an exceptionally large family of phytochemicals found in almost all plants, including food plants. The nightmare vision that threatened to swallow us up was that many more herbs might be banned on similar grounds, but the ridiculous extension to that was, they'd end up having to ban fruits and vegetables too. When herbalists protesting about the change in the legal status of St John's wort cried "unfair" and tried to make a case for leniency, my personal advice was, "Sshh! Don't give them ideas!"

Back to Dublin on the day in question then, a Sunday, if I remember rightly. We awoke to the news that the previous day the health food shop close by had been raided by the Gardaí (Irish police) on behalf of the Irish Medicines Board (IMB). They had taken all St John's wort preparations off the shelves and bagged them up—all the lozenges, capsules, fluid extracts, tinctures and standardised blister-packaged pills.

As they headed for the door the proprietor called out to them, "Hey, what about these?" He pointed to some cellophane bags on the bottom shelf containing loose herbal material with handwritten labels. "What's that?" they asked, genuinely confused. "It's St John's wort tea," replied our friend. Still uncomprehending, the Guards simply said, "We're not interested in that."

When relaying this story in class I am quick to point out that the joke was on them: for my money, St John's wort tea is far more immediately effective as a remedy for low mood than any of the more sophisticated products. As for standardisation, again, I was pitched against a well-known senior herbalist in the *Daily Telegraph* many years ago, in a "debate" on the relative merits of standardisation versus raw or traditionally produced herbal remedies. The *Telegraph* had been directed towards me as, even at that early stage in my career, I had a reputation as a "purist", in Natural Healing terms, preferring my *materia medica* to be as close to fully natural as possible. My senior colleague merely commented that with standardisation, "at least you know what you are getting"—which at the time I thought an extremely odd comment from a herbalist.

Standardisation, or standardised extracts, in herbal medicine, are produced in one of two ways. They may be reinforced, or reinoculated, with an isolated form of their "active principle", to a guaranteed minimum level. Or they may be calibrated by reference to a "marker compound". The marker compound is not necessarily active in any way but serves as a quality assurance mechanism to the extent that if it is found in the required quantity in the plant, it affirms that the plant is medicinally fit for purpose. Standardisation has become quite common in herbal medicine, especially of the nutraceutical variety, and is also the preferred material for use in clinical trials designed to test the efficacy of herbs. In other words, clinical trials on herbs are not usually based upon what might be considered "normal" consumption patterns and contexts, but upon industry standard materials with names like "WS 1442" (Hawthorn) or "EGb 761" (*Ginkgo biloba*).

In my mind this fact gives rise to legitimate concerns about the usefulness, and even the scientific validity, of RCTs[9] conducted on herbal materials and it is necessary, when teaching students of herbal medicine how to read and critique research, to emphasise that such research does not test what happens in a herbalist's practice. What it does test is how a homogenous sample of predominantly male research recruits responds to a pharmacologically controlled substance in a clinically controlled environment. Herbal medicine, and natural medicine generally, is a complex intervention. Not only that but it is individualised according to the constitution, habit and history of the patient. Even if a herbalist did not also routinely give additional health-enhancing advice regarding diet and lifestyle, the remedy itself, frequently an application of polypharmacy—several plants in a "formula"—is itself far more complex than the most sophisticated of molecules designed by pharmacologists (most of them in fact plagiarised from plants in the first place). And even if a practitioner gave only ONE plant as a remedy, that would also be incalculably complex, as any plant you care to mention has not just one, but hundreds of potentially active principles. Herbs have therefore been dubbed "dirty drugs" by pharmacologists: they target too many receptors, in the "lock and key" model of understanding how drugs work. Their effects are therefore incalculable, and of course, according to conventional pharmacology, potentially dangerous. At the same time as being ineffective, of course.

Standardising herbs has been found at the root of some of the most well-advertised allegations of herbal harm or poisoning. The South Pacific herb kava kava (*Piper methysticum*) provides another morality tale. In its cultural context it is a ceremonial plant whose use is deeply rooted in the local community and spiritual life. It is traditionally prepared as a decoction—simmered in water, no additional solvents used, such as alcohol, and there are no medical or health issues arising from its use in those contexts. Medicinally speaking, it is one of the most effective relaxants, anxiolytics and hypnotics in the plant world. In January 2003 the herb was reclassified in UK medicines legislation to "POM"—prescription only medicine—which meant that only registered medical doctors could prescribe it (none would of course, as they are not allowed to prescribe herbs, not having been trained to do so).

The story began in Germany the previous year, when a high-strength extract of kava kava was implicated in a case of liver damage. The suspects were the *kavalactones*, thought to be the active principles in the plant, along with the extraction methods used to optimise lactone content in the product, which employed high-percentage alcohol or even acetone as a solvent. The result was a product that contained abnormally high levels of kavalactones, and none of the buffering chemistry, in particular glutathione, an antioxidant also naturally occurring in the plant, which, in ordinary concentrations, would have protected the liver from damage, but which was destroyed by the solvents used in extraction. Government scientists in the MHRA (the Medicines and Healthcare products Regulatory Agency), in their wisdom, determined that no amount of kavalactone was safe, and took a zero-tolerance stance on the "product" (plant) for the UK market, making no distinctions between different extraction methods despite representations from the herbal medicine profession.

The case of kava kava highlights two important considerations in the regulatory approach to plant medicines. One is that conventional chemists and pharmacologists simply do not understand the ways in which phytochemicals are presented in plants, or, apparently, the concept of *synergy* in plant chemistry—how the constituents work with each other, not as separate agents, but in an interactive, ontological whole. The second—and related—issue is that the isolation of what is effectively a drug from a plant not only misrepresents the plant in its totality but also risks precisely this order of problem—maximising potentially toxic components with none of the natural safeguards. We saw a similar issue related to meadowsweet and acetylsalicylic acid in the previous chapter, with the obvious difference that neither meadowsweet nor white willow got themselves banned on account of their "dangerous" chemicals.

To understand this in depth, however, we need to go to the next level of questioning: why exactly do humans do this? Why do they take from nature, but think that they can improve upon it? Why do they strip away things they clearly do not understand, to end up with a "pure" product? One answer is to be found in the word "product". A product presupposes *sale*, and sale generates profit. Moreover, you can apply for a patent for a product, or a process, which means you can make more money out of it—or, more to the point, you can prevent other people making money out of it without paying you royalties. You cannot patent a plant, and there are few people indeed who got seriously rich selling raw plant material.[10]

A second important element in the marketing of products is packaging. We saw this in the St John's wort story. The advertising and marketing industries have become highly adept in effectively hypnotising their target demographic using visual impact and carefully chosen descriptions. The thrust is to maximise sales. The true goal of marketing is to put products in front of people who want or need them, but as we see so often in advertising, "want" and "need" can also be manufactured and manipulated, or at least amplified, by such practices. It also involves the deliberate down-playing of competitors, done in ways that are perceived as non-confrontational, such as pronouncements that convince buyers that only *their* product has the correct ingredients, patent industrial processing, or indeed the evidence, to satisfy the customer. Believe it or not, this happens in the food and plant medicine world just as much as it does in the white goods or automotive industries. The rosehips that can cure your arthritis *must* be grown and processed using our special methods. Your garden rosehips will not do the same thing. The ingredients that will reverse male-pattern baldness have to be specially selected and processed in our labs: it's no use plastering "ordinary" ginger and rosemary on your scalp. The olive oil with the most effective polyphenols is only grown on our special plantation. And so on and on.

But there is more to this story. In 2023 a regular patient of mine presented with obstetric cholestasis (also referred to as intrahepatic cholestasis of pregnancy, or ICP) in her third trimester of pregnancy. The condition is detected by raised bile acids in a blood test (53 in her case, against a safe maximum of 10µmol/L), is a risk to foetal health and has occasionally resulted in still births. If the condition cannot be brought into balance—and standard medicine offers precious little in the way of validated, effective treatment—the required response is early induction of labour. My client did not want this—or at least she wanted to hold out as long as possible—so she consulted me. I had, in fact, done this before, so without hesitation I prescribed a very simple herbal remedy: dried, cut root of dandelion, prepared in her home as a decoction and taken three times daily. At her next hospital appointment her bile acids were down to 3.

The doctors were astonished, but upon hearing how she had managed this miracle pronounced, "It won't last; they'll be raised again next time." Sure enough they were, this time 52, and the doctors said, "We told you so." My client replied, "Yes, but I ran out of dandelion root. I've got some more now, and you'll see next week the results will be normal again." The following week she tested at 2µmol/L, and at this point the consultant was called in. Having listened to the story he asked for a meeting with me. I met online with him and other members of the obstetric team at University College London and told him what I knew. The possibility of a clinical trial was mooted, to which I enthusiastically agreed, although the consultant was not overly hopeful that the research ethics committee would allow a trial to be conducted using a raw herb and asked if there were—you guessed it—a standardised product that we could use? I don't think anyone has ever succeeded in standardising dandelion root. The trial never went ahead.

I could go on. The problem is, this way of thinking is becoming hardwired into modern human beings—not just scientists, but pretty much everyone, unless they have learned, or been taught, to let it go. The term *evidence* is heavily loaded towards a world-view that measures, analyses, calibrates everything. Subjectivity and anecdote, however remarkable, are at best curiosities, not to be taken seriously in the scheme of things. Standard science, despite its seemingly endless ability to crunch numbers, is not good with complexity: it reduces things (we even refer to it, critically, as *reductionist*) to their basic single components—even though it knows, at some level, that these cannot exist as isolates, but are deeply rooted in whole interacting systems.

Plants resist conforming to restrictive grids. Sure, they obey their own inner directives, but they are notoriously individualistic. In therapeutic terms I tend to emphasise in the classroom that herbal medicine is not a precise science. Attempts to define effective dose ranges, for example, are frequently confounded by individual presentations and conditions—both in the patients and in the plants themselves. Secondary plant metabolites, which in scientific terms form the basis of the therapeutic chemistry of plants used in herbal medicine, can vary wildly from one plant to another even within the same species, according to local environmental conditions. For example, it has been found that the content of thujones in *Artemisia* species is that much higher in plants grown in the Mediterranean areas, such that a normally low-thujone species, *Artemisia vulgaris* (mugwort) may be found to have more than a high-thujone plant, *Artemisia absinthium* (wormwood) grown in the UK.[11]

These are among the more calculable effects accruing to plants, but there are also incalculable effects—although in using that term I'd have to say that to those who *know* plants, they can indeed be relied upon, most of the time. For example, the principle of *amphotericism*.[12] Hawthorn can either lower or raise blood pressure, according to the need of the body. Yarrow will enable blood to flow where it is needed but acts as a haemostatic in case of excess or unwanted bleeding. Ashwagandha may be both a stimulant and a relaxant. A herb that causes abortion in one pregnancy will prevent a miscarriage in another. In such cases the defining principle is the person upon whom the plant is acting, and this implies a complex set of interactions, in biochemical terms, that in effect require a plant to "communicate" with the body in specific ways in order to elicit the correct response. That communication may be explained in terms of receptor sensitivity, or it may be couched in terms of *energetics*, a much more subtle set of descriptors and parameters based upon the character and sufficiency of the vital energy itself.

In making medicines for the market, two things are generally required—apart from that the process of manufacturing should aim to demonstrate appropriate hygiene and consistency. One, the product should be safe. This applies particularly to over the counter medicines. The second is that the medicine should be validated as effective. Interestingly, when the Directive on Traditional Herbal Medicinal Products (DTHMP) was enacted in EU law in 2004, appearing to overturn decades of resistance on the part of the lawmakers in Brussels (who would have preferred to have banned all herbal remedies on grounds of being unregulatable), evidence of effectiveness was not required. Evidence of safety, understandably, was. The Commission took the view that if a product had been in continuous use in the population for a specified time-period, then it could be sanctioned on account of "traditional use", providing the requisite safeguards were in place.

We gave up selling herbal products to the general public in 2005, shortly after the incoming legislation was announced. We had a high street shop, and we saw the writing on the wall. I was always more interested in the plant–people, not the plant–product equation. My teaching career was taking off, and I was away from the shop more often than I was there. The rent was about to go up, so we broke the tenancy and reconfigured our business to prioritise the practice, and the move into education. I still get asked, wouldn't you love to have your own line of herbal products out there? At this I usually educate the questioner by citing the cost of a THR licence (nearly £9K for a single product containing less than three active ingredients), but a more authentic answer would be, "No". With no disrespect intended towards those occupations, I am not a salesman, nor a shopkeeper (I was a truly useless shopkeeper), nor a manufacturer. I might have missed a trick. I do have some wonderful formulations that would probably sell very well. They might afford me an easy retirement and some security for my latter years. But paying yet more money to the government for the right to sell plant products just feels wrong on so many levels.

The decolonisation of plant medicine in our age necessarily goes hand in hand with an upgrade in the ways in which our thought system is structured in relation to plants—along with all natural resources—and will have multiple benefits for our world across many parameters.

The professional practice of herbal medicine contains a fair few paradoxes, and none so cognitively challenging than that which exists between the idea that Nature provides for everyone equally, and the suggestion that the use of plant medicine—and the ability to profit from it—should be reserved to those who have undertaken appropriate training, preferably as closely resembling medical training as possible. The "People's Herbalist" Nicholas Culpeper (1616–1654) resolved this dilemma by using his hard-won Cambridge University medical knowledge to charge the wealthy appropriately for his services, and charging the poor of East London next to nothing, while also educating them in the ways of using simple "backyard" herbs in their own homes. Many herbalists before and since Culpeper have had similar qualms, relieved in similar ways.

The expectation of many prospective patients is that they will find themselves in an arrangement with their herbalist somewhat similar to that which exists between them and their GP. Similarly, the marketplace offers a range of (now neatly registered and accredited) herbal products that mimics a pharmacy, and which are frequently even sold in pharmacies. This model of herbal medicine, a component of the UK market that achieved a gross turnover of nearly £300 million in 2024, and is expected to top £1 billion by 2030, is difficult to get away from. We have been groomed to approve the professionalisation of an ancient healing practice along the contemporary lines of accredited training, clearly defined scope of practice and regulated manufacturing procedures. There is nothing wrong with this *per se*, and we may indeed give thanks for the current UK legislative environment that permits us to practise in this way and facilitates accessibility of our services. However, it may have eclipsed some of the more subtle and arcane dimensions of plant medicine, and it has also legitimised a route for the exploitation of plants under a capitalist ethic.

I am not saying that trading in plant material is automatically and necessarily unethical. I do however offer the opinion that the category of "product" subverts the ethics of healing towards profit; that contemporary technological "improvements" made to plant material for the health market completely miss the point; and that this entire configuration ultimately lacks respect for the ontological status of plants as co-creators of reality. The question I am tempted to ask is, do the plants *mind* this? We must always beware of the temptation towards anthropomorphism, but I was taught from the outset to ask permission of the plants whose help I sought and to take nothing for granted. With an attitude of respect and cooperation, rather than one of exploitation and coercion, I think we can be sure of their assent. They want to participate. They want also for us to bring our medicine in return. My final chapter will address this point.

* * *

For sheer riotous colour there is nothing to beat a bright autumn day in the Northern hemisphere. More so even that the most flamboyant inflorescence of summer. Yellow, gold, orange, ochre and red signal the presence of carotenoids and flavonoids (remember the St John's wort story?) in plant matter—that's why we choose vegetables and fruits with those signatures. It has been hypothesised that the development of the ability to perceive such colours in the first place was an optical biological imperative to optimise antioxidant intake.[13] These colours become dominant as chlorophyll itself decays, revealing the underlying presence of quite other nutrients. They were always there, hiding behind the green, we just didn't see them.

In autumn (Fall, if you are west of the Atlantic), carpets of organic matter gently rot into the ground (if we allow them to), enhancing the soil. Organic matter always acidifies. Minerals alkalise. Plants choose what they need—just like us. It is a time for inspiration, for deep nourishment, enrichment and gestation. The colours themselves move us out of the cool relaxation of green shade and stimulate us,[14] energising, warming and impassioning, providing a charge that can prepare us and take us into, and hopefully through, Winter. As the short, dark days approach we keep the flames of inspiration alight deep inside us.

This in itself, this display of the natural world, is medicine far deeper than the products to be found on the shelves of health food stores, let alone supermarkets. It is however a favourite time to visit the local farmers' market—a treat that lies in store for me tomorrow, as I write this. The produce itself will tell, or reinforce, the story: pumpkins (no shortage of those—or the remnants of them—on the streets today on 1 November), squashes, carrots, parsnips, peppers, apples, berries. There is a world of difference between the words *produce* and *product*. The former implies a process of growing and developing, something alive and energetic. The latter, something finished. Dead?

When I became vegetarian, I was teased about whether I thought plants consented to be killed and eaten. Was I now ethically compromised by this in the same way that I appeared to be about eating animals? I may have lost some sleep—or to put it more accurately, I had some interesting dreams. Giant carrots seeking revenge, pumpkins that could swallow a man whole, toothed leaves that caught and ripped my flesh. Let's face it, there are plants that can kill, and not solely by means of being ingested. Even in the UK, where extreme contact toxicity in plants is rare, handling monkshood (*Aconitum napellus*) without gloves can be extremely risky and has been reported to result in multi-organ failure and death.[15] Was I setting myself up as a target for plant vengeance by picking on them selectively as food?

Obviously, I am employing hyperbole and irony for effect. But what, in fact, are the karmic consequences of eating each other? I am reminded of Eduardo Viveiros de Castro's phrase (and the title of his book) *Cannibal Metaphysics*: for as long as we consign our fellow co-inhabitants to permanent alterity, we may sustain the illusion that we are firstly safe, and secondly superior. But this can break down catastrophically under the impact of natural disasters, accidents and adversity, as indeed it can in the face of our arrogance, anthropocentrism and concupiscence. The decolonisation of the medicine of plants in our age needs to go hand in hand with an upgrade in the ways in which our entire thought system is structured and will have multiple benefits for the world at large. To return to the lesson of elder in Chapter 2, it may serve us to bargain for our lives. We can accept our equality with other species only when we take our place in the food chain itself, not at the top of an agreed (among ourselves) hierarchy, but in the great cycle of physical life, as potential nourishment, in our turn, for someone, or something, else. Someone is always waiting, on some level. We deceive ourselves if we think otherwise.

Notes

1. De Castro, E. V. (2014). *Cannibal Metaphysics*. Minneapolis, MN: Univocal Publishing.
2. *Collins Dictionary* (2025). Available at: https://collinsdictionary.com.
3. University of Essex (2026). Decolonising the library: What is decolonisation? Available at https://library.essex.ac.uk/edi/whatisdecolonisation Accessed 01/09/2026.

4. Waddell, G. (2020). *The Enchantment of Western Herbal Medicine: Herbalists, Plants, and Nonhuman Agency*. London: Aeon.
5. https://www.greekmedicine.net.
6. Burkhari, S. (2024). *The Foundations of Unani Medicine: Principles, Diagnosis and Treatments in Unani Medicine*. Manchester: CUTAM Press.
7. This article in British law was removed in 2004, giving way to the new EU Directive 2004/24/EC, prompting us to give up our high street premises, which in any case were becoming far too expensive. Its sibling, Section 12.1, is still in place (although since the 2012 Human Medicines Regulation it now has a different name) and is the exemption to standard medicines law under which herbalists may still practise in the UK.
8. The figure of £11.5bn was seen in reports, but I have been unable to verify this.
9. RCTs = randomised, double-blinded, placebo-controlled trials – the "gold standard" pharmaceutical trial design, and a lynch pin of what is known as "evidence based medicine" (EBM).
10. There are in fact a few. The first case would probably be the 18th-century American herbalist Samuel Thomson; my own teacher, Dr Richard Schulze might be another. However, these men were driven not by profit, but by the desire to provide effective treatments to patients using naturopathic and holistic principles. In other words, getting rich was not the motive, but an incidental factor.
11. Tobyn, G., Denham, A., Whitelegg, M. (2010). *The Western Herbal Tradition*. London: Elsevier.
12. Amphoteric (from Greek *amphoteros* = both) is a term applied in chemistry to a substance that can act as an acid or a base, depending on circumstances. In herbal medicine it is used to describe a herb that can have opposite effects depending on the needs of the person being treated.
13. See: Jackson-Main, P. (2025). *Natural Healing: Staying Well Naturally in the Modern World*. London: Aeon, p. 82.
14. Lakshmi, V. (2023). Psychological Effects of Colour. *Journal of Biotechnology & Bioinformatics Research*. doi:10.47363/JBBR/2023(5)157.
15. "Gardener dies 'after brushing against deadly wolfsbane flower' on millionaire's estate". *Independent*, 11 November 2014.

CHAPTER SIX

Managing the terrain: gardeners of grace

Consider the lilies how they grow: they toil not, they spin not; and yet I say unto you, that Solomon in all his glory was not arrayed like one of these.

King James Bible, Luke 12:27[1]

The Cambridge University Botanic Garden has been a favourite haunt of mine for fifty years. I discovered it while I was at university here in Cambridge from 1974 to 1977, during which time I frequented it almost weekly. It became part of a walk that I would do every Sunday, starting from my rooms in Churchill College on the Madingley Road, through St John's College and across the Backs, into Sheep's Green and Lammas land, and down into the Western entrance of the Garden. There I frequently spent time in deep contemplation among the plants, in the greenhouses, the walkways and around the lake with its rock garden and causeway, before exiting via the East gate and making my way into town for a meal at one of the three Eros restaurants in either Petty Cury or Free School Lane, drinks in the Eagle, and late-night backgammon with friends in Corpus Christi College.

It was the plants that were the allure of the garden, which sounds unnecessary to say, however in view of what I have noted already about plant blindness I feel it is at least worth mentioning. This was not a mere unthinking immersion in an aesthetically curated version of "Nature": it was a forensic enquiry into the diversity and luminosity of the plant world, undertaken before I had the remotest intention of becoming a "herbalist". I became fascinated by their lifecycles on year-round visits, and although late spring and summer had a special attraction in the form of multiple and often exotic blooms (especially in the glass houses), the other seasons also held sway in their turn through the yearly cycle. I was not particularly handy with a camera—and actually I didn't possess one—so I have no records of these visits. But the visions that awaited me are etched indelibly on my mind to this day, and so are the fragrances. Upon leaving the university, and having chosen the city as my permanent residence, I continued frequenting the garden.

At one point in my life, tired of a succession of temporary jobs pushing paper (or in one case pushing boats on the river), I applied to work in the garden. I had no qualifications for such work, but I thought sheer enthusiasm would be enough to spark interest in me as a prospective gardener. As it turned out I was not wrong, and I landed the job. Sadly, in a way, I had to decline the offer as I had also applied to the food co-operative, where I also succeeded. It was a tough choice between two opportunities, both of which were strongly inviting and very much aligned with my interests and ethics. In the end the job at Arjuna put me in direct contact with the medicinal virtues of plants, and with my future wife.

My relationship with the garden did not end there, however. Upon eventually training as a herbalist and naturopath in the late 1980s and early 1990s, I requested access to the Garden's library for research purposes, in the writing of my qualifying dissertation on *Plantago* spp.—the plantains. It helped on that occasion that I was an alumnus of the University—probably the only serious use to which my degree in English from Cambridge University has ever been put. In that emporium I had encounters with some extremely rare original books—for example, a first edition of Gerard's *Generall Historie of Plantes* (1597),[2] which was easily the biggest and heaviest book I had ever handled: it took help from two library assistants to get it off the shelf, and I had to wear the traditional white cotton gloves in order to turn the pages.

Fast forward four decades and I find myself taking groups of students around the garden on field visits as part of their training as herbalists and then applying for a licence to film educational content there for the herbal medicine course and for the public. These "herb walks" in the garden, both live and filmed, were huge fun to do, not only because they reconnected me with an important part of my past, but for the opportunity that they offered to give back to the plants themselves in promoting their virtues, their qualities, and their long history of association with the human race. Besides that, there are few things in my world that match the excitement of an encounter with a familiar plant ally in the flesh, alive and flourishing.

* * *

The nomenclature of herbal medicine categories is a strange and anachronistic mix of terms hailing from an archaeology of medical usage. We've already encountered the *Alteratives*—a 19th-century conceptual framing of broadly applicable effects that may result in gradual improvement in physiological function across a range of parameters. Added to that, the later addition of terms such as *anti-inflammatory*, *antirheumatic*, or even *antidepressant* rubs shoulders with even more contemporary categories such as *adaptogenic* and *immuno-modulator*. Keen to impress the good doctors of UCL in the story told in the previous chapter, of using dandelion root to cure obstetric cholestasis, I rolled out a wheelbarrow full of what I thought was technical information, only to hear them comment on how much they loved the "quaint" linguistic usages of herbal medicine. I guess that's better than calling it *pseudoscience*.

The *anti-* prefix is especially interesting, since it is after all reflective of a resolutely allopathic approach to medicine. Allopathy, as I have already mentioned, does not have to be the big counter-holistic bugaboo that many take it for, but it does nonetheless necessarily embody some problems, which at least must be talked about. Let's turn our attention once more to St John's wort (*Hypericum perforatum*). Modern colloquial usage has now established this venerable healer as an "antidepressant". As I have elaborated elsewhere (and as herbalists themselves well know), it is much more than that, but because everyone now *thinks* in those terms, not only the terminology, but the *concept*, has become more or less permanently attached to the plant. The term automatically assumes that there is a thing, a pathological entity, called *depression*, but it tells us nothing more about that condition or the people who purportedly suffer from it.

In Renaissance medicine it might have been termed a *hypochondriac melancholy*, but in the 21st century most would almost certainly misunderstand that term to refer to someone whose problem was "psychosomatic". In fact *hypochondriac* means "under the ribcage", and the natural home of the melancholic humour is the spleen—which is located under the left side of the ribcage. The condition arises when an excess of the humour results in a swelling of the spleen and the surrounding area, involving the stomach, the liver, the gall bladder and the duodenum. Anyone who experiences epigastric bloating after eating too much (or even after eating moderately) has an idea of what this feels like. Those who experience a permanent state of congestion and discomfort in the area, a swelling of the upper abdomen, sour eructation and gastro-oesophageal reflux are arguably suffering from the condition, and indeed, according to humoral medicine, one way to give yourself a hypochondriac melancholy is to indulge sanguinity and high living until the excess literally curdles inside you. Traditional medicine has a term for the net effect of this: *stagnation*. Melancholy is the opposite of sanguinity—or the sanguine humour and temperament—but, the ancients tell us, it is the likely destination accruing to its incautious pursuit. So what's that got to do with depression?

Visceral expressions such as *venting one's spleen* ("giving out", as the Irish might say) are the best way to understand this. What do you think happens if the spleen is *not* vented? If the anger, frustration and resentment is bottled up? There is a link here to the liver as well—in TCM the seat of the emotion of anger—and in *The Mind's Eye* I discuss the emotional significance of stagnation in both sectors and organs. There are two entirely functional definitions of depression that do not owe themselves to any narratives involving specific neurotransmitters (serotonin), but take the cue from dynamic, experiential vectors that anyone can understand:

1. The turning back of anger onto the self; anger that cannot be expressed.
2. Knowing what needs to be done but not doing it.

The relevance of the second statement becomes obvious in light of the energetic significance of the liver in embodying our fighting energy. In *The Mind's Eye*, the liver and spleen zones in the iris organ chart are dubbed *The Domain of Assertion*. Assertion—anger reframed—is the fire that enables us to reach for what we want in the world or, conversely, to repel what we do not want. It allows us to set boundaries. Adverse effects in this field of our being may either give rise to unbalanced expressions of anger, or they may paralyse us. Yellow bile, the choleric humour, is anger, but it is also the force of self-assertion; black bile, the melancholic humour, is related to what we call depression, but it is also the natural tendency towards reflection and rumination. There is a direct link. When bile—yellow or black—is suppressed, it becomes stagnation.

I could develop the theme, but I want to say only as much here as necessary to introduce the idea that curing depression is not the simple fix that the term "antidepressant" seems to suggest. St John's wort, in herbal terms, as I have discussed elsewhere,[3] is many things, but above all perhaps, in this context, it is a *hepatic*—it looks after the liver. This is almost never commented upon in standard narratives that discuss its "antidepressant" qualities: that is reserved (as we saw in Chapter 5) for the discussion of the hazards that accrue to its concomitant use alongside pharmaceuticals. To understand how the herb may assist in experiences of chronic low mood requires that we regard the herb in its fullest self-expression. It requires us to consider its role in managing the general terrain of the body–mind, not merely to reduce it to its putative biochemical vectors.

Similar considerations apply to the term *anti-inflammatory*. Inflammation is a natural function of what we call the immune system—although again, to relegate "immunity" to the operation of just one so-called "system" is to ignore the reality that the only system that matters is the overarching biological entity known as YOU. It is interdependent with pretty much all the accompanying "systems"—digestive, circulatory, nervous, endocrine, respiratory, urinary, and so forth. So what, in fact, is an "anti-inflammatory"? Nominally it is an antagonistic and therefore resolutely allopathic therapeutic strategy aimed at suppressing, downregulating or disabling inflammatory responses. The old medical term for drugs used to suppress immunity in cases of autoimmune inflammatory diseases was indeed *immunosuppressants*. Now they are most often referred to as DMARDs—disease-modifying antirheumatic drugs—but the net effect is the same. They come with significant side effects including the exacerbation of other, or even the same, autoimmune diseases.[4]

Inflammation equals pain, one way or another. Pain is indeed a marker symptom of inflammation. The pain attendant upon injury and illness is largely due to the activation of inflammatory cascades that exist to enact the healing. Chronic inflammation, as I have discussed elsewhere, can signal a "failure" to switch off the inflammatory response once the acute phase is over, but it may also indicate the failure to remove the trigger.[5] We don't like pain, so the development of powerful "pain solutions" was always going to be popular.

The single most popular (and profitable) class of over the counter self-prescribed medications goes under the general heading of *analgesics* (pain-relievers),[6] which includes non-steroidal anti-inflammatory drugs such as aspirin and ibuprofen, alongside paracetamol and opioids such as codeine (which is actually PO—pharmacy only—and requires a pharmacist's approval). Together with more powerful medicines only available upon prescription by a registered medical professional, the total UK market in pain-relieving medication is estimated at an astonishing USD 7 billion in 2025, and expected to double by 2035, according to one American market research source.[7] The market for antidepressants in the UK is currently worth over USD 17 billion, expected to rise to USD 27 billion by 2033.[8] Considering only these two classes of pharmaceutical drugs I could comment that we would not appear to be a culture of people who like to *feel* anything very much.

Inflammation can also be "silent", which means that we do not necessarily feel it (or recognise it) but it can, chronically, underlie critical pathologies such as diabetes, cardiovascular disease and cancer, as well as depression and other psychiatric diseases. In other words, we do feel it eventually but, because we typically suppress emergent signals when they arise—and they may arise in contexts that could be regarded as either unrelated or subsidiary, and therefore go undetected in the aetiology of the chronic condition—we can be a long way down the line towards a more serious pathology before we realise what is happening.

Let's look at just one more category in the "anti-" bracket, *antacids*. These are found in two pharmaceutical categories: OTC products, which neutralise stomach acid, and in some cases coat the mucosal surfaces of the oesophagus and stomach to protect against acid erosion; and the deeper-acting proton pump inhibitors (PPIs) and H2 receptor antagonists, which block the production of acid in the parietal cells in the stomach wall itself. They are given for gastro-oesophageal reflux disease (GORD), or in situations where medications for other problems—notably cardiovascular disease—are likely to cause erosion of the stomach lining. In fact, in GORD the problem is more usually LOW stomach acid than high,[9] and reducing stomach acid even further via these medications is unsurprisingly associated with severe nutrient depletion, especially minerals, and can lead to osteoporosis, among other manifestations of malabsorption. You never (I politely suggest) hear people saying, "I've got dreadful malabsorption today!", so this insidious "side effect" is missed, and when it does occur is rarely associated with use of the drug.

Enough has been written on the ill-advised masking of symptoms not to warrant too many repetitions here. The relevance of the cases cited will become clear. The conclusion that I am pointing towards is not so much about how we get it wrong, but how we can get it right. The use of the prefix *anti-* indicates a preference not only for a certain type of treatment (allopathy), but for a view of illness itself as an antagonistic process. As soon as we take on board the fact that the symptoms are NOT the disease, we are in very different territory. In fact we could say that we are forced to engage with the idea that helping the body to do what it is telling us it wants to do might be a better strategy.

When the prefix *anti-* is attached to a plant medicine, I suggest that we need to find a new way to frame what that medicine is in fact doing and move away from pharmacological and explanations and expectations. This necessarily requires us to give our consideration to the terrain and its conditions, and how best to redistribute vitality so that health can again prevail. This is therefore an *ecological* concern. It is about modifying or modulating the *terrain*—the internal environment (*le milieu intérieur*, as Claude Bernard put it). It involves a complexity far beyond the ability of most physicians to calculate—not just doctors, but natural healers too, although I dare to suggest that we may fare somewhat better than those hamstrung by the reductionism of conventional pharmacology.

In the classroom I am fond of reiterating that herbs are not *anti* anything: they are *pro*—pro-health and healing, pro-vitality, pro-*life*. Even where their specific chemistry may offer a degree of threat, that medicine—as we can see evidenced in homeopathy—may still stimulate, promote and support vitality. They do so, as we have seen, in highly sophisticated and complex ways. Where the individual terrain is unbalanced, there may be a number of bases to cover, and this must be done in a harmonious and integrated way, so that we avoid destabilising things further, or pushing the constitution in any exaggerated direction. This in fact comes close to a description of the herbal category of *adaptogens*. Although a problematic category in itself, partly (in my humble opinion) owing to the fact that is not a traditional medicine category and thus overlaps with a more contemporary scientific understanding—which is a problem because science has as yet formulated no clear explanation of how they work—adaptogens are the pre-eminent terrain modulators and cover a range of physiological and energetic bases including adrenals and general vitality, immune response, blood composition, reproductive function, hormonal balance, neurological integrity, digestive potential, nutrient optimisation, and mood enhancement. In traditional medicine they are referred to as *tonic* herbs—*qi* tonics, blood tonics, *shen* tonics *rasayana* (longevity) tonics.

In the right circumstances, however, any herb might be adaptogenic, and many are tonics—they *tone* the system, or parts of it. The word simply means, *to promote adaptation*—to stress, to the environment, to the allostatic load, whatever and however that may manifest. If a specific plant has the right profile of actions to address the physiological needs of any person, then it may act as a stabilising, harmonising agent for that person. The skill of the herbal practitioner is to match the plant to the person. In the case of a single herb, this skill is known as *simpling*—but that doesn't mean it's a simple matter. In fact, it is an advanced skill, requiring in-depth knowledge of a broad range of plants and their actions, as of humans and their pathophysiological profiles. This is also why diagnostic investigations that suit the practice of herbal medicine will elicit far more information than the name of the disease alone can ever give. They will illuminate the various axes, or vectors, across which disharmony may manifest, in patterns that involve interactivity and co-dependency between apparently discrete systems and organs.

A plant, therefore, that is administered as an "anti-inflammatory", may be capable of performing an extremely complex range of immunomodulatory effects—inflammation being in essence an immunological event. The desired effect should never be simply to oppose or suppress, but to harmonise in a way that resolves the inflammation while respecting the body's intention in creating the situation in the first place. This is very different from forcibly switching off inflammation and requires a deep understanding of the underlying dynamics of disharmony.

Taking a herb we have already looked at, the use of meadowsweet in treating inflammation is instructive. We saw that it contains the all-important anti-inflammatory molecule, acetylsalicylic acid, and also that it can act to protect the stomach lining from erosion by that same, or any other chemical or food. It also acts as a mucous membrane tonic throughout the gastrointestinal tract, partly by astringing the mucosa to prevent abnormal leakage. In considering the aetiology of chronic and systemic inflammation, as in the case of autoimmune disease, for example, Functional Medicine tells us that gastrointestinal inflammation leading to permeable (leaky) gut syndrome is a significant factor.[10]

The ways in which plants look after us should give us due cause for reflection. Their "caring" frequently goes to the very heart of the matter, while at the same time addressing co-morbidities and secondary effects, nourishing and protecting key organs, and harmonising the energetic manifestations of what we are pleased to call "disease".

They may also look after our emotional terrain—in fact any therapeutic intervention dubbed "holistic" must always necessarily address this critical layer of health management. This is not only because of the volume of theory that now exists in the field of psychoneuroimmunology, following Candace Pert's famous formulation, *Molecules of Emotion*,[11] which links emotions with physical complaints (but in such a way that we are left in no doubt that the molecules are the most important element in the equation, and still need to be pushed around by other molecules); but mainly because emotions may indeed be, and often are, *primary* in the aetiology of disease. Despite the comparatively recent wealth of scientific data in support of the "body–mind connection", most of us still act as though we *have* a body, and separately, a mind. Emotions are poorly understood, and usually the object of "therapy", itself often essentially suppressive.

Instead, as I articulated in *The Mind's Eye*, body, mind, emotion and soul, or spirit, are all part of a continuum that is an expression of you, your energy-essence, your "higher" self, or whatever else you want to call it. Separation and compartmentalisation—the body itself, the ego, the personality—are constructs that may seem to serve at some very basic level, mainly to facilitate social and occupational needs, but they also act to fragment our experience of ourselves and lend themselves too easily to pathologising—the practice of seeing "something wrong" in ourselves, rather than seeing the glorious whole in an uncritical, non-analytical way that honours our essential integrity.

In particular, we have villainised our emotions. The underlying assumption in the manufacture of "antidepressants" is that emotionality is a problem. People who take them often report that indeed they no longer feel "depressed"—sad, sorrowful, grief-stricken, melancholic: in fact they no longer feel anything. And while it gets them by in the execution of their daily commitments and responsibilities, it is in reality a sort of half-life, a numb and empty existence, a shadow of the life they actually crave. For sorrow is the natural counterpart of joy, and hate and anger of love, resentment and distance of intimacy, and confusion and indecision of confidence, in the morality play of human emotions.

Emotionality is a part of life, and one of our greatest teachers, if we allow it to take its natural course. The clue is in the word: e-MOTION, energy in motion, movement, flow, a cyclical engagement with the deep currents within us, always bringing us back to ourselves. Words and rationalisations are secondary: emotion is primary, and if you watch carefully, it is an *embodied* experience (we don't *have* depression: we *do* depression—it involves posture and attitude). This what the ancients understood in delineating systems of medicine that allocated emotions to specific sites in the body, and in the concept of the temperaments, which were more than just psychological types, but a rounded expression of physicality, emotionality and mentality all in one articulation of the soul.

This is the most cogent reason why a plant can never be an "antidepressant". We have the related concept of *thymoleptic* (mood-enhancing), and a whole range of plants that are classified as such, including but not limited to St John's wort. Traditional Chinese Medicine gives us the category of *Shen tonic*, where the closest English translation of Shen is *spirit*, which, interestingly, resides in the heart not the head. These plants can be better understood in an *energetic* sense, which honours their own unique "personality". But the quest to ascribe pharmacological rationales to their *modus operandi* is doomed from the outset because it is completely reliant on the reduction of the plant's effects to an allopathic molecular equation that somehow must be the precise counterpart to what we think we know about our own "molecules of emotion", and which will usually be chosen to suppress them.

Compare that concept with macroscopic encounters: with the intense bright yellow of the midsummer flowering of St John's wort; with the bluish-purple haze of a field of lavender; with the carnal blush of the Damask rose; with the intricate coronal glory of the passionflower; with the dense white corymbs of hawthorn. We do not have to "take" a plant medicine to benefit from it, but if we do, then what we are ingesting is the totality of effects accruing to the plant—its chemistry, for sure, but also its colour values, its morphology, its affinities with particular organs within our bodies, its folkloric associations and history of human usage, its energetic properties, its psychological and emotional profile, its personality and spirit.

When we expand the field of our awareness to include all available layers of reality—macroscopic, microscopic, atomic, subatomic, quantum, energetic, causal and spiritual—our idea of terrain also expands, and we may recognise that those with whom we share this domain, no matter what species, order, clade or phylum of life, no matter in which level they are focused, all have their role in co-curating our overall experience. And we may then set about the task of choosing our allies and availing ourselves of their specific wisdom.

Molecular reality as we perceive it is not the cause of anything: it is an intermediary level of reality between the "purely" energetic, and the macroscopically verifiable forms that populate what we call physical reality. Dig deeper into it and, as physicists well know, it becomes diaphanous and unpredictable—and, most importantly, receptive to our own intention. When we *coerce* molecules into doing what we think they should do we cut out huge vistas of alternate possibilities that are built into the very structure and fabric of those manifestations. We stultify ourselves and reinforce narratives of determinacy and enslavement. Effectively, we create disease—the experience of being out of alignment. It is a constant paradox that we need form and structure to make life viable, but at the same time we must perpetually dismantle, deconstruct and combust forms that overstay their welcome and become an incarceration.

Causation is down to intentionality, and intentionality belongs to all conscious and aware agents. As humans we are gifted with the extraordinary ability to choose, simply by directing that intentionality towards what we wish to manifest, although few are awake to this possibility. Some might say that we are actively discouraged from it, by education, inculcation, belief and precept. But even in the darkest epoch there are those who manage to find the secret to self-determination. This requires that we cut loose from restrictive governing forms and ideas and forge our own path, create and curate our own terrain. In so many ways, this book is here to suggest that plants are our most familiar, but not always recognised, allies in this task.

* * *

Nature does not need gardens. The physical earth plane is a self-regulating multidimensional energetic field which, like water, always finds its own level, always veers towards equilibrium. But maybe gardens are, after all, intuitive and beneficent, not just to humans but to plants too. In observing garden plants, it has become completely obvious to me that they love being curated and tended by us. Under carefully promoted conditions, they may bloom with added vigour and preternatural beauty. They seem to want to do their best for us. Similarly, when grown for food, correctly approached, they deliver their bounty in spades—pun intended. Perhaps when we garden, we bring out the best in ourselves and in the plants we cultivate? Perhaps we are fulfilling a vital, natural function that has little to do with our cherished "scientific" ideas about Nature, and everything to do with the relationships we forge with our fellow beings, and the opportunities that exist in developing and learning together? Perhaps we are bringing, as I will suggest in my final chapter, the best of our *human* medicine to this planet.

Voltaire's eponymous hero, Candide, after experiencing the full gamut of the dangers and disappointments of the world of human affairs, expresses a simple and empowering truth: *Il faut cultiver notre jardin*—"We must cultivate our garden".[12] We must look after ourselves and those close to us in our orbit, whether human, animal or plant. We must play our part as custodians of the terrain of this earthly reality on all levels upon which it may manifest. And we must do so with the humility and grace of faithful gardeners, letting the plants themselves lead us, as indeed it is the body–mind–spirit itself that leads the plants in the medicine that they offer us.

Notes

1. The King James Bible. (2017). Nashville: Thomas Nelson.
2. The *Generall Historie of Plantes* was one of the first of the great "herbals" produced in the 16th and 17th centuries following the popularisation of the printing press.

3. Jackson-Main, P. (2025). *Natural Healing: Staying Well Naturally in the Modern World*. London: Aeon.
4. The British National Formulary entry for Methotrexate, an NSAID given for rheumatoid arthritis, lists rheumatoid arthritis among its side effects.
5. Jackson-Main, P. (2025). *Natural Healing: Staying Well Naturally in the Modern World*. London: Aeon.
6. Statista.com. (2025). Sales value of over-the-counter (OTC) medicines in Great Britain in 2024, by medicine category. Available at: https://www.statista.com/statistics/415963/over-the-counter-otc-medicine-breakdown-of-sales-in-great-britain/. Accessed 23.11.2025.
7. Marketresearchfuture.com. (2025). *UK Pain Relief Medication Market*. Available at: https://www.marketresearchfuture.com/reports/uk-pain-relief-medication-market-51087. Accessed 23.11.2025.
8. Reports Insights Consulting. (2025). *United Kingdom Antidepressant Market 2025–2033 Analysis Scope: Long-Term Expansion Path*. Available at: https://www.linkedin.com/pulse/united-kingdom-antidepressant-market-20252033-2klwf/. Accessed 23.11.2025.
9. See the discussion in my previous book, *Practical Iridology*. London: Aeon, 2023.
10. Pizzorno, J. & Murray, M. (4th Edition). *Textbook of Natural Medicine*. Elsevier, p. 1771.
11. Pert, C. (1999). *Molecules of Emotion: Why You Feel the Way You Feel*. London: Simon & Schuster.
12. Voltaire, F. (2006). *Candide, or Optimism*. London: Penguin.

CHAPTER SEVEN

Hearing the inaudible music: talking to plants

And those who were seen dancing were thought to be insane
by those who could not hear the music.

Friedrich Nietzsche[1]

I followed the path as it twisted through the wood, penetrating ever deeper into glade and shade, until ahead I saw a dark shape, ivy-covered and mysterious. As I rounded its hulk, I saw a cleft in the broad slab of its rocky side, set into which were stone steps descending beneath its mass. I took the steps, cautiously, as they in turn twisted into the underworld, and as they reached the bottom the space widened into a cavernous atrium, buttressed by tree roots and girded with blossoms, white with a hint of pink.

Approaching me was a young woman in a flowing robe, with a crown of white–pink blossoms on her head, a woodland princess. Her smile was broad and open, her demeanour welcoming. She kissed my cheeks, linked her arm through mine and led me to a door at the back of the atrium, throwing it open to reveal a courtyard strewn with blossoms, with a mature tree in the centre. I recognised it instantly as the source of all the white flowers: Hawthorn.

Carved into her trunk was a seat. I stepped aside, certain that the young woman was going to take her throne, the spirit of Hawthorn merging with her physical form, but instead she ushered me into the seat, and as I sat down I realised that the vista before me had transformed. In place of the walled courtyard was now a wide landscape of rolling hills, soft green meadows and sylvan slopes and valleys, stretching far into the distance. Quintessential England, I thought. I had not seen the countryside this way since my childhood, and I felt a deep longing that took me back to those years, where fairytale and legend were never far away, and when the world glistened with magic and the promise of discovery.

Stirring from my reverie, I became aware that the woman was now seated beside me. I had not realised that there was enough space for us both but understood immediately that such considerations did not apply in this environment. The woman was now older, the youth of her form having given way to mature self-assuredness and command: no longer a princess, but a queen.

We sat side by side for a short eternity, and as I gazed upon this landscape, I felt a charge building in my chest, a volume of emotion that sought to burst through my eyes in floods of joyful tears, and a love so profound that it threatened to dissolve the boundaries of my being into a boundless sea of pure emotion.

After an apparent aeon, the woman spoke. "We must hold the heart-space for this land."

At this, the vision shifted, and I was made aware of great danger from the acquisitive hungry ghosts of disconnected, desacralised human agents with their agendas of fear and greed, and their despotic enslavement of everything free and beautiful, as though they were sucking the vitality out of the land itself in their efforts to assuage the unassuageable. I saw the momentum of this encroachment and the danger that it spelled for everyone in its orbit. I saw the paraphernalia of control—mandate, media persuasion, medication, manipulation—colonising hearts and minds throughout the land, making them fear for their lives and their livelihoods, their domiciles, their very existence, driving them to join in with the endless consumption and destruction, enchanting them with the dark magic of fear, morbidity and malignancy. And I realised that this is what we are all up against, and the dimensions of the ongoing battle loomed large in my mind, causing me to falter and doubt my ability to prevail against any of that. By an effort of will I pulled myself back from the brink.

This, if we are not careful, is the trap that we can all fall into. As soon as we start to think like this, we spin out of the heart-space, and into chaos.

* * *

It was at one of the Plant Consciousness events in London, organised and run by my friends Davyd Farrell and Emma Fitchett, that I met and interacted with the machine that can capture the song of plants, by means of pads that can detect the tiny electrical signals that plants generated in response to a stimulus. Now on sale far and wide under various brand names (and I can no longer remember the precise make or maker—with apologies), at the time this was a revelation to many at the event, and the source of a great deal of excited entertainment, as the plants that had been chosen to populate the presenter stage were wired up to the machine and the speaker broadcast their tunes. To activate the song, we were encouraged to interact with the plants by touching, brushing against them or even just wafting their leaves with the air. The extraordinary thing was that they did not always consent to give their song. Some of them simply would not respond, leaving one wondering what one had done to upset them.

* * *

In case you were not aware of the fact, we are all already dead.

To understand this, we need to understand what death is. If we think of death as a final end to something then this is not going to make any sense, and it may even seem completely insane, demonstrably untrue and perhaps a bit upsetting. However, if we consider plants themselves, we actually use the term "die" or "die back" when the autumn comes around: leaves wither and fall, stems shrivel and harden, and the verdant lushness of the plant world retreats for the winter months. Of course they are not literally dead: they simply withdraw their vitality to a different part of themselves—the root. Even if the plant is an annual—it grows and blooms just once—it has already sent its seeds into the world to create copies of itself in the next season.

The root of our being is not physical. We originate in what some call *spirit*. For spirit, perhaps, read alternative dimensions to the ones we inhabit here in "3D". We are first and foremost spirit, or *energy*, and by some amazing trick that is impossible for us to understand at this level, we transform a part of ourselves into flesh—an avatar with which we navigate physical reality. How powerful is the inner energy essence of each one of us that it is able to perform this trick? Not just create the body once and then wind it up like a clockwork toy to run till it drops exhausted, but to go on creating it minute by minute, second by second, nanosecond by nanosecond, and the same time as constituting through co-creation the very environment in which we live and move. In this the true meaning of healing is found. If you are perpetually creating and re-creating yourself, how and why do you get sick? If you are responsible for the environment around you, why do you find so much in it that displeases you? If you could understand this at the depth from which it emanates, then you could entrain the energy of your body to repair almost any ill and create almost any conducive reality. The implication is that you get sick and experience ill-effects because you are either blocking (or are simply unaware of) your own vitality, or your greater self is sending you a message, or a lesson. Either way it is a situation for learning and progression—evolution if you like. You will probably continue to do it—until you learn not to.

When the physical body dies, we do not go "back" into spirit: we are already there. We are "there" (here) right now, even as the root of the plant is always there no matter whether the plant is in leaf and flower, or dormant—and gestating—in the winter. A part of us that we generally do not notice, or that we actively ignore, never leaves that realm. We may "return" to it often: dreaming is the most obvious route, and in that state, we do indeed accomplish other tasks and undergo other experiences. At death the essence is simply withdrawn from the physical body—much as the vitality of the plant is withdrawn from its aerial structures into the root, leaving the visible body to gently return its elements to the earth. I have already referred to physicist David Bohm's notion that the entirety of physical reality is "blinking on and off", oscillating with imperceptible rapidity between being and non-being—or rather, instead of "non-being", some kind of organising template out of which physically observable effects arise. Bohm refers to this as "the implicate order", and it may have resonances, as we observed in Chapter 3, with Sheldrake's "morphic fields", again an energetic template for the organisation of physical and behavioural phenomena in what we know as "reality". It is possible, in the scheme of our greater existence, that we too are here, and then gone, over and over, throughout hundreds if not thousands of physical existences.

The fact that the idea of consciousness as a "non-local" phenomenon is a rising theme in our current era should give us pause for thought. Fictional, esoteric and scientific literature are all increasingly becoming fascinated with this field of enquiry. In *The Secret of Secrets*,[2] Dan Brown's popular hero, Robert Langdon, hooks up with noetic scientist Katherine Solomon in a characteristic race-against-time thriller set in Prague. In the story, all copies of Solomon's forthcoming book on noetic (parapsychological) research are erased from the publisher's servers by the CIA in a bid to prevent exposing the Agency's involvement in a secret facility deep underneath the city, set up to develop espionage via out-of-body remote viewing, thus weaponising the phenomenon of non-local consciousness.

As we might expect, there have been several attempts to submit the "hard problem" of consciousness to scientific investigation, not merely through the "soft" science of psychology and the behavioural and social sciences, but neurologically, and through the application of quantum principles and hypotheses, in particular, a development of the *Orch-OR* (orchestrated objective reduction)[3,4] theory of physicist Roger Penrose in association with anaesthetist Stuart Hameroff,[5] which proposes that microtubules inside brain cells are capable of supporting orchestrated quantum events to undergo the process of "objective reduction", and suggests that awareness of physical reality is generated as the result of such events being strung together into a continuous stream. The brain is thus likened to a receiver—not the origin of consciousness but its tool and intermediary, continuously translating signals into what we are able to perceive as "physical reality".

Seth, from the esoteric perspective, says something extremely similar in explaining how the construct of physical time in awareness arises as a result of awareness "leaping over the synapses" in neurological events, such that a coherent experience of existence in linear time is produced.[6] And in Bohm's model as well, our perception leaps over the gaps that might reveal the existence of the implicate order, to provide a continuous experience of "objective", exteriorised reality.

The importance of this is that it gets us thinking about consciousness and its relationship with matter—particularly living matter. If we are going to start talking about the consciousness of plants, then it might help to have some way of thinking it through. It turns out that, even though plant physiology is different in several key respects to human physiology, there are resonances. Electrical impulses and hormones—the two most relevant messaging systems used in animal physiology—also occur in plants, although plants do not have a specific structure that is analogous to the nervous system. The question is, what directs these communications, and to what extent can it be said that a plant "responds" to a stimulus that we might provide, other than autonomically (as in some analogue of an autonomic nerve system as found in animals and humans)?

But the same question can be asked about humans too. The mistake here, it seems to me, is in the thinking that conflates consciousness with the essence of an individual. Perhaps consciousness is more usefully seen as a *tool* of sentient beings, one that assists the mediation between an impulse arising in a being, and its eventual expression on any level of reality. Molecular and electrical transfer are also in their turn tools and may represent the lexicon of internal communications within a physical system. That is to say, molecular reality is not a *cause* of anything, but merely the mechanics of the network that actualises the intentions of the individual. Likewise, on another level, consciousness in this analysis becomes a field of articulation, or potential—a milieu in which effects can be produced.[7]

In Chapter 3 I talked about the autopoiesis (self-creation) of a "mind-saturated" universe. In this chapter we are starting to think in terms of what individual participation in that process might look like, and in particular to investigate the extent to which some concept of individuated awareness might apply to plants. When talking of "plant consciousness", however, we may be in something of a cognitive bind, in that the only consciousness of which we have any experience is our own, and therefore we frequently default to anthropomorphic explanations and descriptions. So, in addition to examining the evidence, such as it is, for plant consciousness, we must also consider the problem of translation: how are we going to *know* what plants think or feel? Do they indeed think or feel, in the sense that we ordinarily understand?

When people profess to talk to plants, and more, to receive communications from them, the sceptical position would be to infer sizeable servings of "imagination" from those experiences, which in a contemporary cultural and scientific context would disqualify them from having any standing in "objective reality". It is only in reimagining imagination, or interiority, as a phenomenon capable of carrying truth, that we may come somewhere near an understanding of how these things work. Imagination, as I have said elsewhere in this book, is generative. "It's just my imagination playing tricks on me", as the saying goes, but the real trick is that the universe itself may be the product of a very large and powerful imagination—the imagination of God, if you will. By the same token, our little imaginations may be a whole lot more powerful than we give them credit for.

Researchers in natural science have been addressing the matter of plant consciousness at least since the mid-1960s. Peter Tompkins and Christopher Bird wrote their popular study of plant consciousness, *The Secret Life of Plants*, in 1973,[8] reporting experiments that attributed not only rudimentary awareness to plants, but quite highly evolved telepathic powers and the ability to discriminate in advance when humans bore them, or each other, ill intent. Needless to say, it was quickly served with the tag "pseudoscience" and consigned to the archive of all things hooey and gooey. Subsequently, however, some of their claims begin to look less improbable in the wake of further research.

In Appendix A, I have included a referenced table of key ideas and commentaries on plant consciousness under the categories of science, philosophy, ethnobotany and esoterica. It is not my intention to try and do justice to every researcher and every approach but, through examples that stand out to me personally, perhaps often by reason of my personal history, to summarise the field of available knowledge and theory. In doing so I recommend maintaining awareness of the foregoing discussion on human consciousness, as my overarching contention is that the boundaries between "life forms" as concrete expressions of mind are far less well-defined than we may ordinarily accept. In other words, I want to maintain coherence with the idea of a fluid field of potential out of which individualised forms emerge within the matrix of what we call "reality". Without this, discrete categories risk becoming isolated phenomena, excluded from the possibility of any interaction other than that of an objectifying self-interest. A little further on in this chapter I will propose a model through which to understand that we are all indeed connected in meaningful ways that can be experienced, once we open our minds to the correct method.

A plant-defining legend that arose in my own lifetime is the story of the Findhorn Foundation on the north-east coast of Scotland in

Inverness-shire. In the 1960s, Eileen and Peter Caddy and their three children, along with Dorothy Maclean, having been made redundant by the owners of the hotel they had been managing since 1957, moved to a small caravan park on the barren, sandy soil of Findhorn Bay. Struggling to subsist on unemployment benefit, Peter decided to try and grow food, but it proved a tough environment for humans and plants alike. Dorothy, who had already used her mediumistic abilities to make the hotel business a success, received guidance from beings that she first described as angelic, and later as devas—nature spirits—and was able to give precise instructions on how to manage the small garden. The results proved astounding, exceeding their expectations, and attracting interest from horticulturalists, who were similarly astonished. In time, others came to join them and the Findhorn Community was founded, run according to the spiritual principles given in Maclean's meditations, eventually attracting another spiritual teacher, David Spangler, who would help to establish the Findhorn Foundation, which endures to this day as a centre of spiritual growth, and which in 1975 was able to buy the Cluny Hill Hotel, where Maclean and the Caddys had begun their journey.

The Findhorn story is one of the most impressive, and scarcely deniable, examples of plants and humans co-operating in a highly progressive ecological project, driven by plant intelligence itself, through mediumistic contact involving a sufficiently sensitive human agent. In an age where the food supply itself is increasingly controlled by corporate interests, is routinely produced using intensive farming methods and toxic agrochemicals, and besides that is rising in price year on year such that many low-income families are finding it difficult to subsist, the Maclean/Caddy story should invite considerable interest from anyone engaged with alternative routes to human survival in the face of an inimical and arguably inhuman political and economic environment.

Recent and growing interest in biodynamic farming and permaculture owes much specifically to the work of Rudolph Steiner (1861–1925), the Austrian philosopher, social reformer, esotericist and clairvoyant.[9] Steiner also talked of *Nature Spirits*, or *elementals*, and spoke of the ways in which the spiritual realm (or "supersensible world") interacts with the physical world of consensus reality—the "sense world". He spoke of a 5th-dimensional world, accessible to clairvoyants, where such entities reside and can be contacted by psychically sensitive human beings.[10]

He also suggested that reconnecting with the spiritual world depends upon developing new relationships with these *elementals*—a theme very much echoed in this book.

A key issue here, which I have already alluded to, is that of translation. If we are to communicate with plants, what language will we use? Most of us will, without a second thought, use our native tongue and trust that the "answers" they receive will come back at them in the same manner. There are precedents for this. In mediumship the medium will often make contact with spirit communicators who could not possibly have spoken English during their natural lives, and yet the messages somehow work, and can frequently be validated. Does this point, for example, to an interface in consciousness, a kind of noetic Rosetta Stone, through which communications routinely pass in order to be decoded to the appropriate format?

It turns out, yet again, that there is theory to be accessed in this regard, some of which we have already encountered, Sheldrake's *Morphic Fields*, for example, and Bohm's *Implicate Order*. Figure 4 gives us a possible model for working this through. The *Noetic Field* is the sphere of conscious knowing in which all conscious beings participate, but from within their respective domains. Within that "outer" field of manifestation are nested several other layers governing memory, form and idea, potentially reaching back to original source (*Implicate Order*, or quantum informational substrate), which proceed in direction from individuality to universality, and back in a continuous loop. Translation, or interpretation, can then be understood as a process of sending the thought that you want to communicate to the interior levels of consciousness, where it is decoded and sent back to the recipient as information that can be read within their local noetic framework. From the local to the non-local and back again.

I have devised this scheme to fit the ideas that I want to advance, and it should be noted that the diagram combines theory—or hypothesis—from a few different sources, including the esoteric alongside the "scientific". I am sure that this will provoke controversy among those who believe that the ideas of an eminent physicist (Bohm) should not appear side by side with those of a renegade biologist (Sheldrake, whose Wikipedia entry is an object lesson in what happens to those who do not toe the accepted line in science), much less mixed in with channelled or mystical ideas, but fortunately for the more open-minded reader, I am unfazed by these objections. Likewise, the choice of words to describe

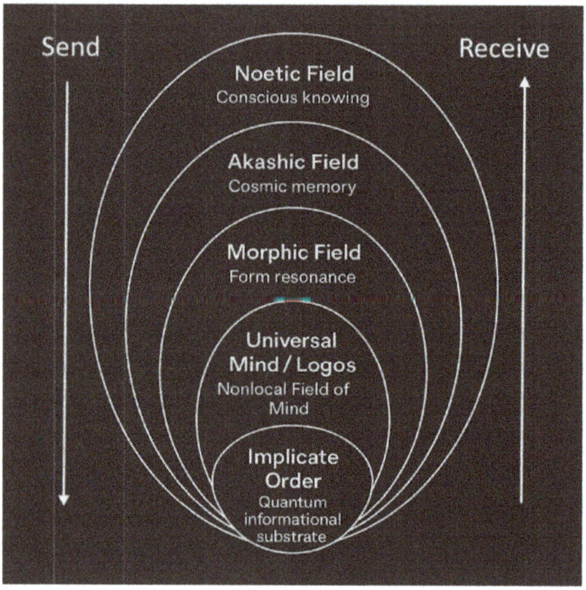

Figure 4. The continuum of consciousness

the various layers, or levels of information. These I have borrowed, or recruited, from diverse discourses, but the overarching scheme I hope can still be apprehended. Let's at least examine the hypothesis and see what it may contribute to our understanding: in fact, shall we just *play* with it for a few moments?

The *Noetic* field: from the Greek *noēsis/noētikos*, meaning inner wisdom, direct knowing, intuition, or implicit understanding. In this level of existence consciousness is "non-local" (not limited by time or space), but it is still definably individual, and subjective. It has also been linked to parapsychology, and phenomena such as telepathy, psychic intuition and mediumship.

The *Akashic* field: sometimes also conflated with the *mental* plane, this is framed as an archive of all events, thoughts and intentions that have happened, or will happen, in the cosmos. It also contains the lexicon which conscious entities draw upon to visualise, articulate and describe their experiences. The experiences of every individual are stored here and are accessible at this level of being.

The *Morphic* field: similar to the idea proposed by Rupert Sheldrake, this level is where the organisational patterns that underlie all forms are generated. Before we can have an individual, or even an event, we need a pattern that gives the character and nature of that individual or event. A cat is different to a dog, a plant is different to a fungus, and so forth.

The *Universal Mind/Logos*: possibly equivalent to the *causal*, or *higher mental* plane in other systems, but it may also reflect the *Buddhaic* plane, and seems to correspond to a version of "heaven"—a world close to the divine source of everything and the natural home of heavenly beings known as *Devas*, which are important in our enquiry as plant and nature spirits themselves are described in esoteric literature as *Devic*.

Implicate Order (Quantum Informational Substrate?): here we might begin to lose the thread somewhat. Multiple searches of the esoteric literature reveal that the "planes of existence" are variously enumerated from 5 to 12—the cutting of the cosmic cake seems not to conform with universally agreed portions. What is beyond universal mind? Can we even begin to ask the question, let alone answer it? In the implicate order we encounter the idea of nothingness as the natural counterpart to somethingness. We encounter the question: "Why is there anything?" The mathematical answer might be framed in the paradox, "A something can exist only when it is nothing."[11] It is the singularity that exists beyond the event horizon, unknowable, unimaginable, uncharted. But possibly foundational.

This system, and the graphic I have presented in Figure 4, may remind some of the esoteric "Russian doll" model of the human energy field derived originally from Buddhist teachings on the planes of existence, which also surfaces more recently in Theosophical and Anthroposophical literature, as well as in the theoretical discussions in the work of Dr Randoph Stone, the developer of the energy-healing system of Polarity Therapy, whose work I have discussed in previous volumes. The names and numbers of the levels are different, and variable, and technically there should be one more level—the outermost (or innermost) circle, the surface phenomenon of physical reality—but the basic idea is very similar, which is that energy, and consequently manifestations of energy such as ourselves, exists on a spectrum of organisational levels beneath the surface appearance, and that these levels are progressively more refined and abstract as we travel inwards, such that we eventually reach levels where we are less individual and more universal in essential nature. At these less individualised levels, we can indeed communicate with quite other life forms and entities, for communication at these levels does not take place through words, or even through thoughts, as we know them, but by means of the transmission of energy impulses, and through direct apprehension—*knowing*—and perhaps even through merging with other individual awarenesses. As Jane Roberts' Seth notes, there are no strict boundaries in what he refers to as psychological reality,[12] no strict division between one soul, or entity, and another.

In practice we do not have to bother ourselves with the mechanics of this: as one medium I asked about the problem assured me, "Spirit handles all of that." We do, however, need to be open to whatever we may receive, and to resist the temptation to rationalise it out of existence because it does not fit into our "normal" conscious ideas of what reality is.

The point is that information exists in strictly *linguistic* form only in physical reality, in the noetic sphere, and to some extent in the akashic, but already exists as other registers of information, or energy, emanating from deeper, more refined and less individualised spheres of awareness. Think about the action of speaking. We string sentences together that add up (hopefully) to a communication of understanding or intent, but where do these come from? We do not have laboriously to "work out" what to say in every case: we trust that once we start talking it will continue to "come out" as a coherent narrative stream. In this way words may well hold more meaning than we generally perceive at surface level. They will potentially carry far deeper intentions and impressions, some of which will be entangled in memory and form (akashic and morphic fields), and some of which may exist in pure syllable and sound as manifestations of *logos*. Sometimes when we are "searching for the right words" we may become aware of a deeper process of investigation into meaning that requires a more nuanced expression, and we will search the lexicon for as exact a co-respondent as we can find, not just to the intellectual meaning, but to the *felt sense* of the intended idea.[13]

In practice all this takes place in a kind of interiority of thought that we may, as noted above, think of as imaginal. Typically, in communications with "plant spirits", the capturing of data registers first upon the mind's ears and eyes, and thus we must become sensitive to the images and sounds presented to us in our reverie or "altered state". Without imagination this is simply not possible. The question of what is "just" imagination, and therefore dismissible, is not a valid one in psychic and mediumistic work, where imagination (the ability to create spontaneous images) is arguably far more trustworthy than the interventions of the rational mind. Practical guidance on the application of this principle will be given in Chapter 9.

Esotericist and occultist Julian Vayne offers the following definition: "Magic is the technology of the imagination".[14] In any case, how do we know, even in ordinary terms, what are the true origins of the interior visions and impressions that any of us may, at any time, experience? As artists, for example, how do we know that the ideas, visions, songs and forms that we create are truly ours, as opposed to signals that we have intercepted and transduced, but that may have originated "elsewhere"? After all, it is only in the physical world, with its concerns about money and survival, that the idea of ownership—or copyright—exists in any meaningful sense.

The native language of plants is first and foremost resolutely visual. As previously noted, there is theory that suggests that our sense of sight itself evolved to interact with plants in ways that mediate our very survival. Of course there is also smell, taste, touch and even hearing. But sight comes first, so much so that in herbal medicine we have the concept of the *Doctrine of Signatures*, whereby the physical form, the colour and shape of the plant, is the intended guide to its medicinal virtues. The colour yellow frequently flags up benefits for the liver (dandelion); red for blood and circulation (hawthorn berries); the shape of the walnut resembles the brain, as do the two lobes of the ginkgo leaf; the micro-perforations in the tiny leaves of St John's wort resemble the pores of the skin, designating that plant as a wound healer; the "thousand leaflets" of yarrow are a visual analogue of the microvasculature of the capillary beds and tell us that yarrow is a medicine that can help where these tissues are compromised. And so on, through many examples.

Smell and taste are also obviously critical in herbal medicine and communicate with our physical bodies in highly specific ways: we have already talked about the bitter principles in plants and their specific actions in stimulating the digestion and toning the heart. Overall, however, what we are considering here is a lexicon that functions at the register of the physical, but which can also allow access to deeper, perhaps less consciously available substrata of our organic, emotional and psychic realities. Bodily organs themselves, as we know from TCM theory, and as I discussed in a previous book,[15] are endowed with emotionality and stand in their energetic reality as placeholders for symbolic aspects of our lived experience, pointing towards lessons that we need to learn, and information that can help us to "make sense" of our lives. The affinity that exists between certain plants and our organic reality can likewise carry significance beyond the physical and can operate to reconnect us through various fields of resonance to a deeper experience of meaning and integration in our lives.

In the more individualised fields, the physical, the noetic and possibly the akashic, we derive meaning from "surface" phenomena—images (including the physical image) and perhaps language—but if we extrapolate to the idea that plants, like us, are "rooted" all the way through the fields to the source, we have a model for understanding how they may communicate with us at far deeper levels—levels where perhaps imagination itself functions as a legitimate part of the decoding mechanism for messages returning through those levels to conscious awareness. It is these strata of translation through image generation, perhaps, that we frequently encounter in folkloric accounts of the plant–human relationship, where plants may indeed take on human characteristics and become the actors in dramas of pedagogy, heroism and redemption—and perhaps even villainy, in some instances. Perhaps we do the same for them?

* * *

Carpets of dayglo pink, electric blue and vivid green demarcate the different zones in the Mind–Body–Soul, OM Yoga, Vegan Life festival, taking place in the decadent splendour of London's Alexandra Palace. Here you may explore multifarious pathways to self-realisation, from the pitch-perfect toning of your bodily flesh in the many bright, Lycra-clad yoga classes; through various esoteric philosophies and meditations; to the purchase of rocks and essences of all denominations. But the plants … the plants in this space are generally, disappointingly, fake. The real things demand altogether too much care and attention in this environment, so everyone brings out the plastic ones with which to decorate their pristine stands: the plant equivalents of mannequins, I guess.

My partner and I usually share a stand here so we can each promote our respective practices, but on this occasion, typically behind schedule with the writing of this book, I am here to support Anji as she navigates the frequency levels, screening out the interference to bring information through for her clients from beyond the veil of the known world, leaving me in charge of the card machine, but with little else to do but keep plugging away at this manuscript. I am making good progress, which surprises me, since I too am surrounded by various denominations of noise—the noise of bustling crowds of festival goers, of deafening and incomprehensible Tannoy announcements, and of shamanic performances that apparently involve hyperventilating, then shouting and screaming at the top of one's lungs into the vast echo chamber of the Great Hall, with its two huge rose windows at either end. Not to mention the psychic noise of hundreds of avid seekers rattling around in their own echo chambers. There is nowhere to escape but inwards.

Or outwards, perhaps. Autumn is in full flight, bright, cold and awash with colour, courtesy of the trees that inhabit the slopes of the Alexandra Park. In a moment of relaxation, I enter "Alexandra Park" in my phone's browser, and I am told that the Park is home to 694 species of plant, 212 species of insect, and 26 types of spider. The Park is rightly proud of its position as the "lung" of North London, and its website boasts scientific studies that validate the ability of green views to reduce stress in just 3 minutes. I think about all the hardworking stress-relievers touting their wares and their patents in this hall, and wonder whether their public might be better advised to save their money and just come to walk through the woods, or join the legions of joggers making maximum use of the air quality to fuel their pumping muscles; or even just hang over the balcony of the South Terrace and enjoy the tree-bounded elevation over the sprawling urban landscape of London for a few long minutes.

But we humans love our interiors—at least, we are supposed to. We are supposed to take our place in the grid, to occupy our square and then fill it with approved stuff: furnishings, white goods, information technology, and, if we are so inclined, the paraphernalia of hobby-craft. Stuff to help pass the time. Stuff to keep us occupied at all costs. So we end up immured, shielded, protected, preoccupied, but perhaps also isolated, in our own Faraday cage[16] of favourite stuff. But not even a Faraday cage is able to screen out all signals, even at the physical level. The Earth's gravitational field, for example, and near-field high frequency signals may still penetrate.

At the root of our being we are always still internally connected through the levels and fields of information, right the way back to the "quantum informational substrate" of the Implicate Order, and quite possibly beyond. These words from Seth seem appropriate: *"Matter is not an imprisoning form. It is a means by which consciousness expresses itself within the limits of the physical field."*[17] We always retain the possibility to travel inwards, there to make contact with whomever we wish—plant spirits, animal spirits, angels, guides: those of our own kind, perhaps, who have, temporarily or not, withdrawn their energy from this field of existence; and perchance also our own "higher" or authentic selves. Some say that in our era the veil that separates us from the "spirit world" is thinning, and that is why interest in the various manifestations of paranormal phenomena is experiencing a contemporary upsurge. It may also be why the forces that are trying to keep us anchored into the matrix are becoming so desperate and so despotic. It is nothing but the tension created by the pulling back of the bow. The arrow will soon fly.

Notes

1. The quote is frequently attributed to Nietzsche, but is not verified. Some say it is simply a popular proverb.
2. Brown, D. (2025). *The Secret of Secrets*. New York: Bantam.
3. Penrose, R. (1989). *The Emperor's New Mind*. Oxford University Press.
4. Penrose, R. (1994). *Shadows of the Mind*. Oxford University Press.
5. Hameroff, S. & Penrose, R. (2014). Consciousness in the Universe: A Review of the 'Orch OR' Theory. *Physics of Life Reviews, 11*(1): 39–78.
6. Roberts, J. (1994). *The Nature of Personal Reality: Specific, Practical Techniques for Solving Everyday Problems and Enriching the Life You Know*. San Francisco: Amber Allen Publishing.
7. See: Varela, F. J. & Maturana, H. R. (1980). *Autopoiesis and Cognition: The Realization of the Living*. Dordrecht: D. Reidel.
8. Tompkin, P. & Bird, C. (1973). *The Secret Life of Plants: A Fascinating Account of the Physical, Emotional and Spiritual Between Plants and Man*. New York: Harper & Row.
9. See: Steiner, R. (2004). *Agriculture Course: The Birth of the Biodynamic Method*. Rudolph Steiner Press.
10. Steiner, R. (2016). *Nature Spirits*. Rudolph Steiner Press.
11. Hockney, M. (2016). *Science's War on Reason*. Self-published.
12. Roberts, J. (1994). *Seth Speaks: The Eternal Validity of the Soul*. San Francisco: Amber Allen Publishing.

13. "Felt sense" was a concept popularised in psychotherapeutic literature by Eugene Gendlin in his 2003 book *Focussing: How to Gain Direct Access to your Body's Knowledge* (London: Rider). It is framed as a way of bringing non-verbal experience and knowledge into awareness and anchoring it via an appropriately resonant linguistic handle.
14. Vayne, J. (2026). Personal communication.
15. Jackson-Main, P. (2024). *The Mind's Eye: Personality and Behaviour as Revealed in Quantum Iris Analysis*. London: Aeon.
16. A Faraday cage is an enclosure constructed to block electromagnetic activity. Made from a mesh of conductive material, it acts to diffuse ambient electrical fields and waves within its structure, thus leaving the interior free of interference. It is used to protect sensitive electromagnetic equipment from external radio frequency interference (RFI).
17. Roberts, J. (1964). *The Early Sessions, Book 2*. New Awareness Network, Inc.

CHAPTER EIGHT

Encounters with the master plants

Hail to the Star of the North
Daughter of the flower of Jurema
When we embark on our journey
May she be our guide.

Amazonian Icaro[1]

"I want to go and see this shaman," said Anji one day. "He's just opened a shop in the Grafton Centre. I met him the other day and he told me to drop by and see him." "OK ..." I said, doubtfully. I wondered what a shaman was doing opening a shop in a mall, but I was well-used to the instincts of my wife and from experience I judged she probably knew what she was doing.

The "shaman" was what we might politely describe as "a piece of work". He was American and had a sharp, acquisitive eye that he turned onto my wife in a look that I had long learned to recognise as predatory. He paid me no mind at all. I wondered whether it was her money or her honour that interested him most—or perhaps both. The shop was a poor copy of establishments that in a previous age we used to call "head shops": a range of incense, crystals, diaphanous textiles, small boxes inlaid with mother-of-pearl, and of course the obligatory hash pipes, "skins" and gauzes. At the first opportunity I managed to persuade Anji that enough was enough, and we managed to get away from this unimpressive man and his emporium.

No sooner had we regained the street than we—almost literally—ran into a friend of ours. Jane had shared various adventures with us previously: on one occasion we all took part in a Reiki apprenticeship that turned out to be run by the Angel Gabriel and Mary Magdalene. It was a source of huge hilarity in later reminiscences, so when she ventured, "D'you wanna come to a ceremony?" we agreed unhesitatingly. She turned to her side and for the first time I saw a small man with swarthy dark skin and a long black ponytail under a wide-brimmed leather hat. "This is Tchydjo. He's from Brazil." The man looked over at us, and I caught a glimpse of coal black sparkling eyes in an otherwise expressionless face.

"He's a shaman," continued Jane in a matter-of-fact tone, as though it were an everyday event.

As we left the encounter I whispered to Anji, "You do know what we just agreed to, don't you?" She looked back at me. "What? It's a ceremony, right?"

* * *

I am mesmerised by the whirling and swaying of the Pajé. He sings as he drums, of the King and Queen of the forest. The grandfather and grandmother. I intuit the reference to the Vine of Souls, *Bannisteriopsis caapi*, and the chacruna leaf, *Psychotria viridis*, the principal components of the Amazonian entheogenic brew known as Ayahuasca, or *Yagé*. It is about 40 minutes since we all ingested the brew, and the effects are starting to accelerate. So much so that I have that familiar sense of needing to focus on the song, the *icaro*, or risk losing myself in the rapidly spinning maelstrom of kaleidoscopic visual effects. Bizarrely, this time I am getting garden tools—spades, hoes, rakes and shears—diving and wheeling in fast motion, a thousand perfect replicas of themselves, but the colours, the colours are disgusting, rank, putrid, nauseating. I inevitably succumb, and the retching feels like I am being turned inside out. I taste the brew coming back up and reflect for a lucid moment on how the medicine has already entered my bloodstream, so losing the residue will make no difference. But then the fear, gripping and insistent, a perpetual and bottomless reservoir of horror that seems to be rooted in the very basis of physical reality.

I have seen it before, and it is the reason why, time after time, I wonder why I subject myself to this process. And then I know. The dam breaks, the stomach is emptying itself, again and again; where does it all come from? The small glass of sacramental decoction that I swallowed could have been refilled a hundred times with what is coming out of me. And as the physical liquid is expelled, I have a powerful sensation that I am being purged emotionally too. Every pore in my body is expelling the dark residues of stagnation and putrefaction, both physical and energetic, and I am bathed in hot sweat. I recognise the effect of *la medicina*, and I am content, even while having little sense of who, in fact, *I* am in this intense moment of fragmentation and reduction. I begin to breathe deeply, to relax, to let go into roller-coasting currents of pure joyous energy, and it seems as if the dance of the shaman is physically driving those currents, pushing them around and around, inviting the beneficent spirits into the mix, while somehow dispelling the mischievous and maleficent ones. As he does so he utters swooshing noises, interspersed with imitation birdsong and underpinned by the rattle, a contraption of gourd, seeds and feathers, shaken in a hypnotic triple-time swing that evokes deep memories that I can't quite identify, something ancient, something primal, something that penetrates into the farthest reaches of my ancestral memory, something that seems to have the power to reach deep into my DNA and whisper, "Time to find out who you really are …"

The garden implements have given way to far brighter visions now. I seem to be on a plateau, surrounded by preternaturally coloured blooms and small beings who scurry and labour around me, apparently keeping everything in order. They are unconcerned by me and I resolve to let them do what they need to do. I am aware of the hard ground of the forest floor beneath me, and at the same time I know it is not hard, or solid at all, in fact: it is not really there. I am suspended, cradled and buoyed up by a web of pure light that seems to extend both inside and outside of whatever it is that I call "me". I am aware of a deep radiance that seems to be just outside of my field of vision, and at the same time is in me and of me. I am falling into the light, sucked in, tumbling in hysterical laughter, weeping and crying, my head now threatening to cleave in two, and suddenly the shaman is in front of me, his face painted with strings of white dots that seem to draw my focus back towards earthly reality. He was mid-song: "*Ela seja sua guia*!" He places his hand on my solar plexus and with a swoop I am back. "*Bom*?" he enquires solicitously. "*Bom*", I reply, gratefully.

From there on we work. Work, in ceremonial terms, is completely interior and can be gruelling. It is the downward slope from peak experience, a long, gliding, cyclical journey, wherein portions of my reality continually present themselves to me, almost as if asking to be reworked, rethought, reframed, reimagined, along no particular logical timeline. I have the sense that I may go anywhere, fly, visit remotely people who are important to me. My mother calls and I am aware of a pain in my chest. She has recently been diagnosed with a regurgitating aortic valve. I feel the ancestral heart, struggling with its long burden of guilt and shame, and I know that my path as a healer is bound up with that. I know that that is part of the deep pain I am called to work with. I know I carry it. "Born with a weak heart/I guess I must be having fun"—I explode with laughter and tears of pure joy as the words of the Talking Heads song slip into my mind.[2] I send healing—and love—to my mother, and I know she receives it. I know that my difficult relationship with her is redeemed in the fulness of time, perhaps accelerated by this journey. I see her father behind her, applauding me with his eyes. He died of a heart attack in his 60s—about my age as I participate in these ceremonies. I am said to be very like him. I send healing to both of us.

Words and phrases form in my mind, and I have a sense of the urgency to remember them: they may become the handles that enable me to grasp what the ceremony was "about" once the mind, no longer given wings by the medicine, returns to baseline consciousness. I can feel that possibility coming closer, the words spiralling around my head more insistently, trying to capture, to contain, to preserve the experience and its meaning.

Suddenly however, the shaman, who has been quiet for a while, allowing us to work in the deep silence and stillness of the forest at night, arises and starts to move again. Swoooosh. Shoooooo. Wheeeeeee. Schwit-tchwoooo. He begins his dance anew, wheeling and gyrating with his arms held wide and his face upturned to the night sky, and I feel the energies stirring, the mind-bending effects of the medicine start to gain in intensity again, and I realise, incredibly, that he is doing this, with his movement, with his utterances. For the Amazonian curanderos and curanderas, the medicine is not wholly contained in the brew, with its chemicals and molecules as Westerners believe, but is ushered in by the spirits themselves. To myself I mutter, "Oh no, don't be starting that again, please!" But another part of me is secretly excited and anticipatory for what comes next.

This reignition, this restimulation, may happen three or four times during the course of the night, and at a certain point the shaman will inevitably get up again, holding out the flask containing the herbal decoction and tempt us with, *"Um pouco mais?"*—"A little more?" This as we all know, separates the sheep from the goats, the men from the boys and the women from the girls, and not many are minded to decline, no matter that we know the whole exhausting scenario is going to run and run all over again, from the dizzying, nauseating merry-go-round of the upwards spiral, to the work-filled interdimensional spaces. It is necessary to develop a great deal of stamina to join ceremonies such as these. They are not for the faint-hearted in any dimension.

At the end of it all, in the intensification of the darkness that takes place just before the dawn, I am flat on my back, wrapped up against the penetrating cold in layers of blankets, staring up into the canopy of trees, sleepless amidst a gentle symphony of snoring—including that of the shaman, now wrapped in his sleeping bag with his partner beside him. I had tried to sleep. I could not. I closed my eyes and curled up in my thick carapace of blankets, hoping that sheer exhaustion would carry me away, but there was nowhere to go. My mind was a-light with spinning luminescence, spinning visions, spinning words, a sort of existential vertigo, round and round, falling and being caught again and again. Somehow the very notion of sleep itself seemed absurd. Something whispered to me, "The Spirit never sleeps". I turned onto my back again and allowed myself to stare open-eyed into the branches once again. Geometric patterns took over, each fractal a cosmos in itself, constantly evolving and developing, generating worlds and trails of significance that spun off to follow their own existences. Suddenly I seemed to be in quiet conversation with the Great Spirit Itself, as It reminded me gently, "You will sleep soon. I cannot. Look at what I am holding. Look at what I am generating every nanosecond. You are here because I do not sleep. I hold you and all of creation in the cradle of my thought. You are made of me. You can trust me not to drop you or forget you. Now sleep, my child."

* * *

A vital role of the *shaman*[3] in ceremony is to guard the portals of the ceremonial space so that the spirits he or she wants are invoked, and those that might disrupt, or whose medicine is too strong, are kept at bay. In this way they hold the space for everyone, and in the context of a ceremony, are immediately and acutely aware of everyone's state. They are often also expert *vegetalistas*,[4] knowing not merely the outward form and character of the plants they use, and not necessarily being expert in the preparation of the medicine (this in Amazonian terms is the business of the *Ayahuasqueros*), but knowledgeable about their spirits, their intentions towards humans, and the means by which they may assist the work of healing.

Once again, for transparency, I am not attempting to rewrite any theory about Amazonian shamanism or usurp the territory of ethnobotanists or other researchers. I write from my own experience, from what I have gathered in association with one such healer, and as a herbalist—a *vegetalista* in my own terms—as well as out of my own fascination for the plants themselves, their energetic reality, their personality, and the agency that is imputed to them through narratives such as the one I am presenting in this book.

The term "Master Plant" arose out of the interaction between "Westerners" (I prefer the term *Europeans*) and the native Americans of all tribes. In the context of the indigenous cosmology, each plant has its place, but we in the Europeanised world love our hierarchies. In truth, the Master Plants may be regarded as the kick-ass teachers, but not everyone needs their ass kicking. Most of the European persuasion probably do. So when a plant comes around and kicks the shit out of us, in some apparently perverse way we enjoy it, and we go back for more—often missing the point, as we are apt to do. Sometimes it can take quite a few kickings to empty us of all that shit. If indeed it ever does.

Please understand that I am not recommending these practices or advocating them. They are not comfortable, and there are other pitfalls unseen by many in their eagerness to receive *la medicina*. I was lucky. Tchydjo is one of the kindest, most compassionate and most committed healers that I have ever met in any context. He had been handed a brief by his own elders to bring the Medicine to Europeans. Many Amazonians are engaged in similar missions, aware that the very fabric of their traditional lives is in danger from the aggressive encroachment of the European love affair with imperialism, colonialism and consumption. They need us to understand what is at stake, what could be lost if we do not curb our insatiable greed and concupiscence. What better way than to engineer an encounter with our very souls?

But some practitioners (of all denominations) are less than kind. Some are themselves disciples of "self-service". They are after fame, money, power, and influence, and they are not afraid to use their advanced powers of perception and magic to promote those personal aims. I am not saying this is wrong. It is complicated. All humans, wherever they come from, may share the same range of emotional possibilities and preferences, no matter that in some cultures these may have been institutionalised. I am saying *caveat emptor*—buyer beware. If you ingest a poisonous plant, there is a strong chance you will be poisoned. It is the same with some humans. They are who they are. In their own way, these too may be medicine, as previously discussed. It is up to us to avoid and stay out of trouble—or to navigate and understand the reason for our involvement, if we get caught up in that. It is up to us to develop our own knowing in these matters. The Master Plants are not the only plants who can help—or protect—in this. This is why in the next chapter I will invite you to consider and choose your own plant allies, and I will offer you suggested methods of doing so.

Usually included under the umbrella of "Master Plants", and in some understandings exclusively referred to by it, is the ethnobotanical category of the *entheogen*. The word means "generating the divine from within", and these agents are also variously referred to as psychedelic (mind-producing) or psychotropic (affecting the mind and causing changes in mood or thought patterns)—although to be clear, the latter category also includes psychiatric drugs alongside "recreational" or ceremonial substances.

Two issues arise from this: one, the categories of "recreational" and "psychiatric" suggest an order of allowability in terms of social acceptance of these two seemingly different practices, but the true distinction is between self-medication (recreational drugs *always* function as such, which is different from saying that they are advisable), and conventional, state-sponsored medication. In debates on reforming "drug laws", what frequently comes to the surface is that governments make no money from the sale of street drugs. Watch the debate on cannabis very closely, and you will observe what has happened to this plant. It is now available to us on medical prescription for the treatment of certain "conditions". But it is no more available to us as a legal substance (maybe a replacement for alcohol, which is arguably far more dangerous) than it has been since the original (UK) outlawing in 1928.[5]

Again, I am neither promoting nor deprecating the use of cannabis. My friend the Brazilian Pajé, noting that young people in his community had begun to use the plant "recreationally", took it upon himself to ban it for his own people, not because in European terms he considered it immoral to "get high", but because he saw it as disrespecting the plant itself. In his *materia medica* cannabis was reserved to a very specific purpose—the relief of menstrual pain. This is especially interesting from a "Western" scientific perspective, where it is known that the plant has significant phytoestrogenic effects.[6] Perhaps this traditional medicine man was able to see far other dangers than the ones broadcast to us in the anti-cannabis propaganda? In my own youth I was a prolific user of cannabis. It did me very little good, in fact it virtually paralysed me; it took the fight out of me. It was a trap from which I struggled for years to escape. I am fond of joking that the lawmakers may have missed a trick in banning it, rather than licensing it. A more docile and ineffectual population can scarcely be imagined than one "high" on cannabis.

However, in the "developed" world, we are required to pay duty to the powers that be if we want to change our minds in novel and emancipatory ways. In other words, the state is not concerned about the harm that you may come to in using these substances, which in many cases is far less than that accruing to the use of licensed pharmaceuticals, but about the fact that you place yourself outside their jurisdiction. As Graham Hancock convincingly argues, it is no accident that substances that are capable of radically altering your very perspective on life and its priorities are heavily targeted by the ideological state apparatus. He is talking about regimes of control that do not want us to know who and what we really are, and what we are truly capable of.[7]

The second issue accruing to the categorisation of psychotropic drugs is that some of the most powerful mind-acting pharmaceuticals available to medicine are still directly extracted from plant material. Surprisingly, in contrast to the discussion in Chapter 3, wherein we saw that drugs that were once based on naturally occurring molecules are now synthesised from petrochemical byproducts, opioid drugs are still largely dependent upon the cultivation of *Papaver somniferum*—the opium poppy.[8] These include morphine and codeine, as well as other more powerful analogues such as heroin (diacetylmorphine), whether manufactured pharmaceutically or produced for the black market.

Although the opium poppy is commonly associated with areas such as Afghanistan, where it is typically cultivated for the black market, its natural habitat is in fact the Middle East and the Mediterranean area, and the overwhelming portion of supplies destined for the pharmaceutical industry come from Palestine (75% in 2022), Serbia and North Macedonia.

The story with the Andean plant *Erythroxylum coca* is not dissimilar. Prized by both the pharmaceutical industry and the black market alike, coca has an uneasy relationship with the global human community, no matter that in its own geographical area it is an important medicine, as a general tonic, digestive stimulant, and a specific remedy for altitude sickness. The tropane alkaloid extracted from the plant, cocaine, gives the starting material for benzocaine, novocaine and lidocaine, variously effective as local anaesthetics and anti-arrhythmia medications. Its recreational use is notorious for enabling extremely bad human behaviour the world over, not least in its geographical area of highest distribution, where it provides the basis of a significant black-market economy worth an estimated $100 billion.[9]

Seeing these effects, I find myself wondering what the intention of these plants is in appearing on the planet and interacting with us. Is their dual nature—poison versus cure—part of a conscious plan, as such, or merely an impersonal device that operates to inflict automatic punishment on those who would use them inappropriately? Or is that even a difference? The natural custodians of such plants rarely have issues with them, and yet, once in the hands of "Westerners" they seem to start generating problems for us. We saw that in the case of kava kava (Chapter 5).

Perhaps the premium example of this dynamic is *Nicotiana tabacum*—tobacco. If you want to talk about Master Plants, then throughout the entire American continent, North, Middle and South, the indigenous people hold this plant, above all, as sacred. It is the chief ingredient smoked in the *chanupa* (peace pipe) of the Lakota and many other tribes; it was integral to ritual and magical use in the Mayan culture; and it is used in Amazonian ceremonies to provide protection for and prepare those about to enter the sacred space: *"Tobacco smoke envelops the body of the person as a protective veil, pervading its smell and awakening a state of alertness."*[10] On the website of *Takiwasi*, a non-profit civil association, located in the city of Tarapoto in the Upper Peruvian Amazon region, appears the following statement:

> *The reductionist mechanisms of positivist–rationalist thought lead to the profanation of the spiritual dimension of all authentic healing acts and, especially in the case of tobacco, they transform this remedy into poison. Tobacco, "powerful mediator between humans and gods", may play an essential curative role, particularly in psychotherapeutic processes and in the search for answers to the pressing existential questions of modernity.*[11]

"Powerful mediator between humans and gods" is a very large remit to fill, and echoes the material presented in the foregoing chapter. Tchydjo's medicine circles, not only those concerned with Ayahuasca but others that I attended, such as the *Padroes* ritual,[12] were routinely prefaced with a tobacco ceremony. A large smudge-stick of cured leaves was placed upon a shovel and set alight. The shaman and his assistant would approach each member of the circle in turn, wafting the smoke towards the aspirant with a large fan made of feathers, while singing prayers of intention for the ingestion of the medicine.

The practice of smudging itself is highly interesting. In North American tribal tradition it is often done with "sage", however, on closer investigation, although in some cases herbs of the *Salvia* genus are indeed used, very frequently the "sage" is actually an *Artemisia* species, usually one of the handful that go under the common name of *mugwort*—which itself is a magical herb of considerable significance, and is also used in the acupuncture practice of moxibustion. There is more "science" than might immediately be obvious behind this ritual, and usually resolutely spiritual practice. Smoke penetrates—deeply. It enters crevices and orifices from which even water would be barred. The antiseptic properties of smudging alone validate it as a cleansing and purifying practice.

I met Linda Black Elk, ethnobotanist and activist from the Lakota nation, at one of the *Plant Consciousness* events at Regents Park in London. I was suffering with a horrible affliction of the upper respiratory tract at the time, which I was having trouble shifting, so I asked her if she had anything on her stall that might help. She told me that she would normally recommend tarweed (*Grindelia camporum*) but that her supply had been confiscated by the UK Border Force (shades of Dr Schulze's experience described in Chapter 5). I said, that's lucky, as I have some at home. But then she said, "Also take this", as she handed me a hard, black lump of the polypore fungus *Inonotus obliquus*—chaga—with instructions on how to prepare it. I went home and did as she had suggested, and in the space of a couple of days the "infection" was greatly reduced but not gone. On the Monday we were booked for a more select workshop that she was giving with her husband, Luke Black Elk. She asked after my health, and when I reported that her advice had worked, but there was more to do, she said, "This will finish it", and smudged me with chaga. By the end of that short day all my symptoms were gone.

Since "giving up tobacco" as a one-time cigarette smoker I have ingested tobacco via ceremonial smudging, via the pipe, as the powder *Rapé* blown directly into my nasal cavity, and as a ceremonial tea. I cannot say that I have enjoyed those experiences very much (except the smudging, that was always good), but I can vouch for its potency, and I can fully accept the proposition suggested to me that as a previous abuser of the plant, I may have to pay a price in order to get to know it more intimately as an ally. The story is told that, when the indigenous people saw the Conquistadores imitating their tobacco-smoking practice, they noticed that the Europeans were inhaling the smoke. Alarmed, they rushed to correct the habit, but the Europeans thought they knew best—or suspected that the natives were trying to hide something important from them—so they kept on doing it. Eventually the locals gave up saying, "OK, let them discover why not for themselves!"

At the bottom of all of this are two vital thoughts. One, the injunction to respect the plants themselves at the deepest levels. Linda Black Elk, again, talks of her "plant relatives", emphasising kinship, not difference. And two, the necessity to respect those who know the plants best and are qualified by virtue of their long association with them to teach others their ways. In particular, the untutored use of powerful ceremonial plants is more than inadvisable: it is also arguably arrogant and stupid. In addition, Ayahuasca tourism, the phenomenon whereby unsuspecting visitors, usually of the European persuasion, are lured into ceremonies by operators of dubious quality and intention, may be taking an unacceptably high toll on the physical and mental health of participants, as also upon the cultural heritage of the indigenous people themselves.[13]

Meanwhile in the "West" we are making molecules again: lysergic acid diethylamide tartrate 25 (LSD) derived from a fungus (ergot) that grows on cereals; mescaline, a powerful alkaloid derived from the San Pedro and Peyote cacti; psilocybin extracted from *Psilocybe* mushroom species, the alkaloid ibogaine from the African plant *Tabernanthe iboga*, and of course dimethyltryptamine (DMT), the "active" molecule in Ayahuasca, in combination with the harmine alkaloids that act as monoamine oxidase inhibitors to prevent the molecule being metabolised before its active effects can be fully experienced. All these substances have been subjected, over several decades now, to rigorous scientific trials to assess their potential as medicines—particularly psychiatric medicines—and have been found effective in the treatment of anxiety, depression, addiction and even psychosis.

So, what's not to like? At this point that is something of a revision question for those who have come thus far in this book. Reading Rick Strassman's classic of psychedelic literature, *DMT: The Spirit Molecule*,[14] I am mainly struck by how much I would *not* like to participate in such experiments. First, I have formed the clear impression that there is a fundamental world of difference between research-grade DMT and the sacred medicine of the Amazonian cultures. The latter is a piece of indigenous technology deeply informed by the spirits of the plants themselves and administered by expert spiritual leaders and guides. The former is a clean, but clinical, substance administered and monitored by people who are 1) not participating in a commensurate manner and 2) may have no knowledge whatsoever about the deeper dimensions of what they are doing: they are after all "researching" it—which in itself tells you that they may not yet know anything worthwhile. This is not an entirely untutored perspective: I have ingested most of those molecules at various points in my personal history.

This habit, the necessity to test to destruction remedies and medicines that are millennia old, in order to construct our own grid of "evidence", and by doing so establish (or not) their effectiveness and safety according to our generic Western standards, is a peculiar addiction of the developed scientific world, and one we have seen and critiqued previously within these very pages. It has threatened to kill traditional medicine in Europe and elsewhere, and it militates towards the twin pillars of control and profit. It therefore stands in diametric opposition to almost everything I am proposing in this book, which sounds very absolutist and possibly intolerant, but is in fact simply a personal preference and choice with which you are welcome to disagree.

But I do not want this chapter to be solely concerned with the psychedelics. In my mind the term Master Plants may direct our attention towards some rather different possibilities. If we are to go with my suggestion that plants have agency and are expert in recruiting other species to work with them in mutually beneficial ways, maybe we can go further and suggest that the true "masters" are the entities who have developed this symbiotic skill to "Master's" level—or beyond. I call them the global plant superstars, and they include many "common" medicinal plants—in fact the more common the better: dandelion, nettle, elder, yarrow, St John's wort, wormwood, mugwort, to name but a few of our local heroes. I regard all these individuals as Master Plants.

All herbalists get into patterns of prescribing, and I am no different. I have often thought about this and wondered if it is laziness or lack of imagination. Then I reflect that in every case, these are the plants I have learned to trust, and on whom I can rely on to do the job I need them to do. I know of a herbalist in Ireland who grows all his own herbs, but typically only engages with a dozen or so in his therapeutic interventions. This is not ignorance: it is the product of a profound and intuitive knowledge, and relationships that have been forged over many years, and perhaps also passed on from previous generations, giving him unprecedented depth of understanding of their potential as healers.

I have also noticed that the further and deeper my relationship with the plant world goes, the more I can respond to the intuitive dimension in prescribing. When I worked in the Lancashire practice, Abbotts of Leigh, I strongly felt the presence of my predecessor, the late Charles Abbott, standing behind me in the consulting room, guiding and approving my choices. It made the whole process of seeing people in that unfamiliar context easier and more confident (I am a soft Southerner and could frequently feel myself something of a stranger in East Lancashire). As time passed, I suppose because he had trained me to his satisfaction, he came less frequently, and I began to notice that it was the herbs themselves that stood around me ready to jump in as needed—and they still do. I get this particularly with astragalus root, a herb from the Chinese tradition (also much in demand in typical TCM formulations, by the way). Occasionally, when the herb suggests itself yet again, I ask the question, "Isn't there someone else?" The response is almost indignant: "Why are you looking for someone else? Aren't I good enough?" "Well, I just thought, you've been doing a lot of work lately: wouldn't you like to delegate?" Again, the reply is dismissive. "Just get on with it. You know it makes sense."

* * *

The oldest yew tree in the UK—possibly in the world—is found in the churchyard of the village of Fortingall in Perthshire. At an estimated 5,000 years old, it is by no means the oldest tree on the planet, but it is possibly the oldest non-clonal tree in Europe, meaning that it is still supported by its original trunk. The root systems of the Norwegian spruce, *Picea abies*, commonly used as a Christmas tree in many cultures, have sometimes reached nearly ten thousand years but these are clonal trees—although they spring from an ancient root system, the individuals themselves may be far younger.

The age of trees generally is a fascination for a species whose individuals typically live somewhat less than a hundred years. Trees have witnessed the history of humankind over centuries of change and development—our battles, our defeats, our triumphs, our technological advancements, our philosophical, political, and possibly even our spiritual growth.

The yew itself (*Taxus baccata*) is a regular denizen of graveyards, where it was placed, some say, to deter animals from grazing on consecrated ground, on account of its extreme toxicity (see later). Others say that thriving on corpses made its wood especially strong and pliable for the making of weapons (longbows) and musical instruments (human cadavers do indeed, apparently, make high quality fertilizer). However, the narrative that I personally prefer is that Christian churches were often sited on ground that was important to the earlier pagan religion, which was a way of recruiting—or coercing—those from the Old Religion into the New—the Christian. To the pre-dating pagan religion, and especially to the Druids, the tree symbolised both mortality and immortality—the ongoing cycle of death and rebirth. It was the portal to the underworld, as it was the Rainbow Bridge to the Otherworld. In modern syncretic narratives it is also said to "anchor" the angelic realm upon earth, although the tree functioned as the *Axis Mundi*, or World Tree, forming a bridge between the three realms—Earth, Underworld and Otherworld—long before angels entered the discourse in these Northern lands. Some say that the great tree of Norse legend, the giant ash *Yggdrasil*, was in fact the yew—although I'd say that there is no harm in leaving this to the ash, as each tradition has its own preferential relationship with these beings. There does not have to be just one *Axis Mundi*.

Churchyard yews are usually kept in a typically cropped status, their upward thrusting branches appearing almost to defy gravity in an inversion of what many might see as a "natural" tree shape. Left to its own devices, however, the branches of the tree travel over in an arc towards the ground again in toroidal fashion, taking root around the tree to generate new trunks, and forming a womb-like space under the canopy of branches around the central trunk. The trunk of the tree itself, over hundreds of years, may also subdivide, creating a second hollow space inside the very heart of the tree. Yew-shaman Michael Dunning reports spending over nine years in the "sanctuary" of this space, and in doing so recovering from life-threatening physical disease and receiving initiation into the sentient spiritual and healing wisdom of the yew.[15]

The yew and the elder often grow together. In the cemetery close to where I live there are several individuals whose branches are literally entwined with each other. Elder is similarly a tree whose folklore reaches into the afterlife, and the transport of souls from the earthly realm to the Other World. The two together form a powerful alliance, but I do not mean to suggest that this association with death is a negative connotation—either for the yew or for the elder. That is not my experience at all, as I will witness below.

But there was a second event similar to the loss of our elder hedge described in Chapter 2. On this occasion a well-established border between our land and our neighbour's contained a variety of shrubs and trees, including ceanothus, laburnum, jasmine, ivy and yew. It grew to a height of around eight to ten feet and was an effective and familiar boundary. Hedges make good boundaries especially because they are generally porous: they do not completely block either vision or sound, but they do hold space, and they make a conducive backdrop against which to relax and enjoy one's natural space. This one also served as a habitat for wildlife—birds, butterflies and bees, in particular.

Then one day our neighbour, equipped with an armoury of gardening tools and herbicides, and altogether unannounced, started to systematically destroy the hedge along the entire length of the garden. Granted, it was "his" hedge—meaning that his was the legal obligation to maintain the border on that side of our garden, and granted, most of it was rooted in "his" soil. We pleaded with him, but to no avail. "It's my garden, I'll do what I want", was the reply. We tried to plead the cause of the bees, in particular. "Nasty things, bees, they just sting you", came the rejoinder. We could only look on in horror as these beautiful friends of ours, plant animal and insect, were massacred and banished for good.

One consequence of this was that the plantation of ornamental acers (maple variety trees) that were our neighbour's pride and joy, no longer had any substantial competition on the plot, and started to grow unfettered, very quickly reaching unsustainable proportions and threatening to overshadow our entire garden unless cut back: it has of course been left to us to look after that job on an ongoing basis. Human ignorance and stupidity are my downfall when it comes to practising tolerance and forgiveness. We retaliated by erecting a six-and-a-half-foot solid wooden fence down the entire length of our garden, and just a couple of inches inside the border ("it's our garden: we'll do what we want"—but to be fair, we also had an obligation to ensure that our dogs did not escape and run riot over the neighbourhood).

It was the loss of the yew, particularly, that I mourned. I had literally just discovered the tree in my own Plant Spirit training and had been overjoyed when I realised that we had one as a companion in our own garden. As part of our training, we had made an essence of the yew berries. The physical medicine of yew is deadly poisonous and is contained in almost all parts of the plant—leaves, branches and wood, and the seed-kernels, or cones, of the berry. However, the gelatinous, preternaturally magenta, sweet-tasting flesh of the berry, in which the cones are enveloped, is the only part of the plant that does not contain the potent cardiotoxic taxine alkaloids, and which may be eaten quite safely, once the cone is removed. Taxine alkaloids form the starting material for the chemotherapy drug paclitaxel, marketed as Taxol.

The *dieta* with yew, however, did have a most remarkable and powerful effect on me. Several hours after the ingestion of the yew essence and having almost forgotten the lesson of the day and its associated folkloric and historical significance, I retired to bed. The room we had been given was unusual in that it was in fact pitch black in the dead of night, having only one "window"—a small skylight, invisible from the bed itself, that fed a small amount of light into the room during daylight hours, but which at night, especially in the absence of any lunar effulgence, rendered the room opaquely dark. Waking in the very small hours, around 2 am, I found myself staring up into the darkness and being enveloped by a richly textured dark green luminescence that seemed to envelop me and whisper comfortingly to me. The texture and the shapes of the leaves and branches were instantly recognisable as those of yew. It was not unlike my experience under the canopy of the forest in the medicine ceremony described earlier in this chapter, and although far gentler and less challenging, it was every bit as vivid and remains as powerfully with me to this day. It seemed to reflect an eternity of plant–human association, and bestowed a level of peace, stillness, wellbeing and safety that I have rarely experienced, before or since.

Notes

1. *Icaros* are ritual songs sung in Amazonian *vegetalista* ceremonies. This is my translation from the Portuguese of an *icaro* that was routinely sung in ceremonies I attended with Pajé Tchydjo of the Kariri Xoco tribe of North-Eastern Brazil. Jurema is *Mimosa tenuiflora,* a mildly hallucinogenic plant used ceremonially either alone or as part of the entheogenic brew, Ayahuasca, in that part of the Amazon.
2. Talking Heads. (1983). This Must Be the Place (Naïve Melody). From *Speaking in Tongues*. Sire Records.
3. The terms *shaman* and *shamanism* strictly speaking apply only to practitioners from Northern Asia, and derive from the Russian word, *šamán,* which was originally applied to the traditional healers of the indigenous people of Siberia. Over the past few decades it has been annexed to refer to practitioners of any indigenous spirituality practised in navigating the spirit world for purposes of divination or healing.
4. *Vegetalista* is the name given to Mestizo shamans of the Peruvian Amazon. These practitioners believe that they receive their knowledge directly from the plants themselves.
5. https://en.wikipedia.org/wiki/Timeline_of_cannabis_law.
6. "Apigenin, the aglycone of a flavinoid phytoestrogen found in cannabis, displayed high affinity for the estrogen receptor." Sauer, M. et al. (1983). Marijuana: Interaction with the Estrogen Receptor. *The Journal of Pharmacology and Experimental Therapeutics,* 224(2): 404–407. Available at: https://pubmed.ncbi.nlm.nih.gov/6296360/. Accessed 23.12.2025.
7. Hancock, G. (2015). The Consciousness Revolution. In his *The Divine Spark: Psychedelics, Consciousness and the Birth of Civilization*. London: Hay House.
8. The Royal Botanical Garden at Kew. (2025). *Papaver somniferum: The Opium Poppy*. Available at: https://www.kew.org/plants/opium-poppy. Accessed 23.12.2025.
9. Eser, A. (2025). *Cocain Statistics*. Zipdo. Available at: https://zipdo.co/cocain-statistics/?utm_source=chatgpt.com. Accessed 23.12.2025.

10. Mabit, J. & Giove, R. (2012). *Sinchi, Sinchi, Negrito: Medicinal Use of Tobacco in the Upper Peruvian Amazon.* Available at: https://www.takiwasi.com/docs/arti_ing/sinchi_sinchi_ing.pdf. Accessed 24.12.2025.
11. Ibid.
12. *Padroes* translates from the Portuguese simply as patterns, but has other connotations, especially regarding patterns of ancestral energetic affiliations that might be holding us back in our spiritual development. The ceremony was essentially a cutting of the umbilical cords of attachment pertaining to our ancestry, and a freeing up of our spiritual energy for our own healing and for our creativity.
13. Shipibo healer Pedro Tangoa López shares these concerns in an impassioned essay, which can be accessed here: https://medicinadelsol.com/dangers-of-ayahuasca-tourism-maestro-pedro-tangoa-lopez/.
14. Strassman, R. (2000). *DMT the Spirit Molecule: A Doctor's Revolutionary Research into the Biology of Near-Death and Mystical Experiences.* Rochester, VT: Park Street Press.
15. Dunning, M. (2025). *Yew Shamanism.* Available at: https://yewmysteries.com/the-yew-mysteries/. Accessed 27.12.2025.

CHAPTER NINE

Finding your plant allies: a magical practice

> *... you consider yourselves above a plant, and do not realize what a fine consciousness they possess*
>
> Seth[1]

We had been in our garden a few years before one day it occurred to us that we had no nettles. Nettle is not only a signature medicine plant in Western herbal practice, being an alterative, nutritive, antiallergic and antirheumatic (immunomodulatory), as well as an adaptogen, but also an extremely important spirit plant ally, associated as it is with the martial energy of protection and assertion. It is sometimes likened to a Roman Centurion: tall, upright and dangerous, not to be crossed. This connection may also have something to do with the story that many believe, following statements by the 17th-century British herbalist John Parkinson later declared to be false, to the effect that nettle was brought to the British Isles by the Romans, who used its sting topically to relieve the effects of a cold, damp, rheumatism-inducing climate.[2] However, while it is possible that they did indeed bring their own species, *Urtica pilulifera*, there is archaeological evidence to support the idea that the common stinging nettle goes back at least to the last Ice Age in the British Isles, and possibly to the one before last.[3]

It is, however, ubiquitous and abundant in contemporary times, and we had never before had a garden that was not at some point colonised by the plant. It seemed that no sooner had we formed that thought in our minds than we noticed a nettle patch against one of our border fences. We spoke kindly and appreciatively to them, and they appeared to flourish for a short while, before mysteriously sickening and dying. We suspected poisoning, as we had seen the plants on either side of the fence, and our neighbours on that side (the other side to hedge-destroyer) had small children. We spoke to the plants and suggested that next time they arrived they place themselves well inside the border. Sure enough, a few weeks later, a second crop arrived, again seemingly out of nowhere.

To those who will say that I am romancing here, I will grant the following concessions. Plants propagate their seeds in a number of ways, including being spread by animals and insects, and simply blowing in the wind (anemochoria). Nettle is described as a "pioneer" plant: it will typically move in and colonise bare and unused ground, but usually it spreads through seed dispersal in the immediate locality. To us, however, it seemed oddly significant that, although technically it could have arrived at any point—or even been there from the start of our own occupancy—it chose to arrive at the moment we acknowledged its absence. Or perhaps, our acknowledgment itself was a communication from the plant announcing its imminent arrival?

Observing nettle in the wild reveals a typical tendency of the plant to grow as a border, around the edges of woods, along pathways (probably spread by human footfall), and most interestingly, encircling single trees. I visited a solitary oak on a broad hillside in the Quantock hills, growing at some distance from nearby woods. In my quest to sit down within the folds of its trunk at ground level I had to penetrate a thick circle of nettles, which precisely demarcated the canopy area of the tree. It was as if the nettles were protecting the tree, acting as a barrier to prevent unwanted invasion. The sting of the nettle is indeed a deterrent to the unwary and to those who do not take steps to befriend the plant. However, as mentioned above, there are those who have used even the sting for medicinal purposes, in the treatment of arthritis and rheumatism.

Medicinally, nettle has powerful "antihistamine" activity, which is to say that it can help in allergic afflictions. Interestingly, in traditional Chinese medicine, allergies are often framed as "external invasions of wind". Wind is the only pathogen in TCM that originates outside of the body itself, so once again the motif of protection against invaders can be intuited. Among allergic conditions, the plant's Latin name, *Urtica dioica*, gives us the name *urticaria*—nettle rash. The name derives from the Latin word to burn—*urere*. (In fact there is a related species with a far more virulent sting that bears the name *Urtica urens*—the "burning, burning" plant.) Nettle rash is an allergic affliction and is thus an example of the ways in which plants can signal their actions through their various physical properties, not just appearance, but other impressions that they invoke, in this case both physiological and sensory.

The second part of the Latin name is *dioica*, which means "two houses". It refers to the fact that the plant is *dioecious*—it has both male and female individuals, and both are needed for its propagation. This is in contrast to a *monoecious* plant, where the male and female organs are located together on the same plant. These features will be discussed a little further on in this chapter, as we get to grips with the gendering of plants, but in respect to the nettle I have noticed that students express strong views on whether they visualise the plant as male or female. One of our students wrote her graduating dissertation on nettle as a herb for facilitating pregnancy and childbirth. To her, nettle was self-evidently female. Many, however, choose to go with the martial aspect (the Roman Centurion) and, ignoring that martial qualities can also be carried by female individuals, impute the male gender to the plant. Does it matter? Guidance will be given further on in this chapter!

* * *

Establishing a basis for practice

In this chapter we are going to get practical. I do not want to dumb anyone down, but the basic principles of forming conscious relationships with plants are extremely simple, and do not need to be complicated. Remember "plant awareness disparity" mentioned in my Preface? The first step is to begin to *notice* plants, to include them in the range of experiences and conversations that you permit yourself to have day to day. Plants are already aware of you: you are simply returning the favour. If you are already somewhat aware, you can build upon whatever baseline you currently hold and expand it. You do not have to embarrass yourself by making this socially obvious—unless you want to. The silent, internal acknowledgment of your plant neighbours, cohabitors and co-creators is usually enough.

I recommend that you make an inventory of the plants in your life. It doesn't have to be exhaustive. You will find there are far more than you could probably have imagined prior to doing this exercise. Don't overwhelm yourself. They may be houseplants, garden plants, food plants, medicinal plants. You might find yourself focused particularly on textiles or furnishings. Anything goes in this exercise, but try to come up with a manageable range of individual plants that you can start to explore.

Then begin to inform yourself about these plants. Writer Stephen Harrod Buhner recommends not knowing too much about the plants you want to communicate with, as "facts" external to the plants can take over and influence your impressions. If you agree that this might suit you better, you can skip to the later section in this chapter where I suggest a practical platform from which to communicate. However, I personally enjoy finding out about the plants I encounter. I find it enriches my relationship with them and adds meaning and depth to the association—especially finding out about folkloric and cultural associations, which gives information about the history of that plant's pre-existing relationship with the world of humans.

It is worth installing a plant identification app on your smart phone. It is true that in the early days these were not 100% reliable, but as with most technology, its human inventors and guardians are generally motivated to increase accuracy and efficiency in successive updates, and I am aware of far fewer issues than used to be the case. Correct identification of plants can be important for a couple of reasons. Firstly, it means that you can confidently pursue deeper research by working with the precise species that you are interested in; and secondly, if there is a safety issue, for example with toxicity, you are better placed to make an informed decision as to how—or if—you want that relationship to develop in the future. If you are interested in actually ingesting the plant, and are otherwise untutored in plant medicine, this is a must.

If you want to develop your plant relationships in a healing capacity, my strong recommendation is that you work with a suitably qualified professional or even go about getting yourself trained. This does not have to be a full professional training. There are several courses offered at domestic level, such as the *Herbs for Everyday Living* course offered by the UK college for which I teach.[4] Studying herbal medicine is one extremely powerful way to start building meaningful and intimate relationships with specific plants and working with them practically in your day-to-day life and that of your family. I do however offer the following advice for such studies:

- Although you may study a wide range of plants, select a small range of your favourites to hold that little bit closer to you. Maybe even choose one or two to go deeper with. The structure of the professional training that I administer is such that students are enabled to take a deep dive with individual plants that catch their imagination in the form of specific graded assignments. This also enables them to hone their research skills and develop the ability to discriminate between good information and bad.
- If possible, either grow, or find growing wild, the plants you choose to go deeper with. Get to know their life cycles by direct observation. Visit them often, in the wild, in your garden, on your windowsill (you'd be surprised how many people have houseplants that they manage to ignore for weeks on end).
- If you want to use plants for medicinal purposes, do them the courtesy of preparing them yourself, with love, gratitude and awareness. Don't default to "supplements". Get to know their taste, smells, how they respond to traditional preparation methods, and what these methods add to their efficacy.

Above all, take regular walks in the open air in areas where plants are foremost. Even in cities you will find parks and greens, trees and border shrubs, and—once you start really looking—all kinds of small and seemingly unassuming individuals poking up through cracks in the tarmac or between the layers of bricks. Take an interest. Stop and say hi. Use the plant recognition app (or a good wildflower identification book) and find out about them. Take the research home and go deeper with a few chosen reference books (see the bibliography at the of this book), or even via online searches. Find out how these plants have already impressed themselves upon human awareness and what they have already contributed. Even if the plant is already familiar, beware of just accepting your prior knowledge as all there is to know. Make the effort to find out more. The next time you meet them you will know each other better, there will be instant recognition—and usually a profound and growing sense of connection the more you hook up together.

Since becoming a herbalist, walks in the open air—city or country—have become far more interesting and loaded with added significance and opportunities to learn. In the early days do not swerve from using technical assistance in identification: you will need it less frequently as time goes on. Likewise, inform yourself of the folkloric aspects and the cultural resonances of the plants you come across. Eventually, if you are so minded, you will start to forge your own communications, and ideas and knowledge will come through more direct channels.

A beneficial "side effect" of all this is that you will also become far more attuned to the natural cycles of the earth and its seasons. We have constructed an environment in which we can just about function without having to consider this too much: from front door to car door to office door and back again, central heating automatically adjusted to follow ambient temperatures, all year round with little distinction. If we do have to contend with "weather" it is often accompanied by a grim clenching of teeth and voluble complaining. Remember there is no such thing as bad weather: only the wrong clothing, as the Norwegian proverb has it. This is one reason why my partner and I refuse to buy a house without a chimney and an open fireplace or wood burner. We use central heating as rarely as possible, and we frequently throw open windows, even in zero temperatures, to freshen our environment and prevent the stagnant fug of an enclosed human habitation. At the very least have plants inside your houses: houseplants have been shown to improve air quality and even strengthen the immune system.

Lastly, never forget to offer your thanks and gratitude for all that plants do for you. You may be sitting on a chair right now made of wood. The chair may well be covered with a padded seat of plant origin. You are also very likely wearing clothes made of cotton or linen (or even nettle, bamboo or hemp); and you will (unless you are on a strict carnivore diet) almost certainly be eating plants within the next few hours (and even if you eat animals you are still benefiting from the plants that those animals have already eaten). And when you retire to bed at night you might welcome the comfort of cotton or linen bed sheets.

Lastly, if you are reading this book from a hard copy, as opposed to a digital download, the very pages upon which you focus are made of specially prepared wood pulp known as paper.

Of course, there are modern synthetic alternatives to all—or most—of this, but these often come with unexpected health and safety warnings, and in my view are generally *just not as nice*! Original fibres and textiles, original and traditional building materials where possible, and a predominantly plant-based diet are the non-negotiable baselines of my own habitual preferences. And I am eternally grateful for all of that. So what is the exchange? What do we give back in return, apart from grateful thanks, perhaps? Am I not just consuming, once again? Maybe, but consumption is, after all, unavoidable—as I hope has been adequately discussed in the foregoing chapters. Mindfulness, however, is its own gift, and an essential commitment; and in addition to that, to support original and traditional industries that grow and use plants, as opposed to large-scale commercial exploitation for profit, is increasingly seen as proactive in guaranteeing sustainability on all levels. Properly, sustainably managed, biodynamic and organic plantation, agriculture and forestation are going to be essential in rectifying many of the ecological—and possibly also the *economic* problems that we face today.

Preparing to dialogue

In Chapter 7 I suggested that our ability to communicate with plants is natural and self-evident once you concede that we occupy and inhabit not just the same physical dimension but have also other levels of existence in common. I also indicated that we don't necessarily need to be aware of the mechanics of how it happens, and that "imagination" may be all we need to make it happen. This is a basic principle of magic, which has to do with the adoption of an alternate theoretical framework in which the customary dependence upon logic and verifiable fact may not apply—at least not in the way we usually think of it. Remember that we are trying to get away from all that, rooted as it is in assumptions that in themselves have led, over the last few centuries, to significant distortions and abuses, and have arguably landed us in some particularly hot water—to go back to the analogy of the frogs in the cauldron.

So, the first step, please, is to *suspend disbelief*. English poet Samuel Taylor Coleridge talks about *"that willing suspension of disbelief for the moment, which constitutes poetic faith"*. Poetic faith, in his terms, is *"analogous to the supernatural, which stimulates the mind's faculties regardless of the irrationality of what is being understood"*.[5] Although I have already dealt with the concept of the "supernatural" (nothing can be "super" natural: it's all just natural, only some of it may not have been "discovered" yet, in orthodox scientific terms), I do resonate with the idea of the *magical*, and the basis of magic is different from the psychological orientation we are used to. In magic we can make our own rules, with our own imaginations, for what we want to happen, and trust that anything we can imagine is probably true, or at least possible. Too much picking apart will simply result in a squalid mess of doubt and indecision. We do not have to "understand" it, in intellectual terms. One might say, we need a holiday from that!

In fact, magic also has logic, but it is not the logic that we know and understand, the logic that we have been taught to follow and obey unquestioningly. Seth calls it "Framework 2"[6] (Framework 1 is the normal, everyday logic that we routinely rely on) and explains that it follows a different logic which, although we have been taught to mistrust and even reject it, is equally valid. In fact, it may be more psychologically native to us than that which we later acquire as a result of schooling and inculcation and perhaps represents a far more primordial manner of apprehending the world, one which perhaps can still be encountered in childhood, and in communities that we have marginalised as "primitive". To access it we may have to give up our precious attachment to rational logic, "common sense" and reason, and make space for something else to happen.

I suspect that if you have come this far with me in this book you may at least be considering this as a possibility. It has something also to do with the proposition cited in Chapter 1, that you cannot solve problems with the same mindset that created them. We already arrived at the basic understanding that something's got to change, in our thinking, in our attitude, in our belief system, in our approach to the world. What have we got to lose?

A better question, in relation to the subject matter of this book, is, how can making friends with plants help us, individually and as a species? I hope the answer is at least starting to become obvious. By "making friends" I do not just mean the applied acquisition of "facts" leading to further exploitation and colonisation that we mistake for knowledge and culture. I mean learning how to co-construct a reality that is amenable to us both. The fact that we don't currently know what that may look like is rather the point. We need first to render ourselves impressionable to the *ideas* of other beings. We need, in effect, to *listen*.

So, we are going to start with listening. Take a look around you. Where are the plants? Are you indoors? If so, do you have houseplants, or at least cut flowers? Or are you outdoors? How are plants contributing to and shaping your environment? If you can't see a plant, find one. Any plant—but pay attention to the quality of your attraction to whichever plant you eventually choose. Next, I invite you to feel stupid. Firstly, in that you are about to talk to a plant. And secondly, that you may be about to learn something that you don't already know. You may want to be alone for this. You don't have to admit to it afterwards. But you do need to comfortably suspend any scepticism and disbelief, at least for a few moments.

Next, become still, calm and receptive, and allow the physical reality of the plant to register on your senses. This can include, for the time being, its visual appearance and its smell. For touching and tasting we need to put some cautions in the mix—refer to my previous comments about educating yourself. For listening, we are going to move into a different kind of psychological space. Try to regard the plant with appreciation: tell it what you like about it. Remember the experiments referred to in Chapter 7: plants respond to our emotions and to our intentions towards them.

There was a much-publicised experiment in which two identical plants were made available to schoolchildren, who were instructed to lavish praise and appreciation on one, while reviling and insulting the other. You can guess what happened: the appreciated plant thrived, while the insulted plant withered and died. I do not recommend you repeat this experiment, which like many such initiatives is rooted in an alienated, dispassionate, not to say cruel mindset, but it does demonstrate that plants are not oblivious to our intentions.

Make sure that your plant knows that you do not intend harm, and that you are willing to learn from it. You can speak your intention out loud if you want, or you can just say it in your head. It makes no difference. Once you have made this introduction still yourself again and listen. Pay attention to anything that pops into your mind, without judging it, dismissing it or explaining it. Preferably note down what you receive.

Then you may ask some questions. These again can be spoken out loud, or simply "imagined" in your head. It doesn't really matter what kinds of questions you ask, but it might be best to start with the kind of thing you might ask a human that you are meeting for the first time. You would not, probably, go to the deepest existential levels at the first encounter. You would be more likely to enquire, "Where do you come from?" or "How are you today?" Then simply listen to the answer. Give it time, and accept whatever comes, even if nothing does. Accept the nothing as an answer in itself. Remember the device for listening to plant song, also from Chapter 7: the plants did not always agree to participate. Do not judge this eventuality, or take it personally, but be receptive to whatever enters your mind from this point. It may not be verbal, there may be images that arise, feelings and sensations. If words do come, note them without judgment or filter. You may not immediately understand them—don't expect that plants will necessarily think the way you do. There is abundant space for the symbolic, the poetic. Allow a few minutes for the conversation, and then respectfully withdraw your attention.

Take the time to write down what happened. Be honest and faithful to the actual experience, don't elaborate or interpret. Simply note it. This is because you may not fully understand it at first, but if you relate the raw experience, rather than your hastily interpreted version of it, there is a greater chance that you will be able to retrieve the meaning later, when you have time to reflect on it.

Asking permission and negotiating exchange

My strong recommendation is that you practise simple conversations with plants before trying anything more demanding. When harvesting plants, for example, I was taught from the very beginning that permission needs to be sought. Remember the invocation to the elder in Chapter 2: an exchange is suggested. At the very least we owe it to these beings to consider not only what they may do for us, but also what we can do for them. Most of the time the simple acknowledgment with gratitude is enough. The experience may be significantly deepened by this very simple gesture, but it is a gesture that needs to be practised.

Before picking a flower or a herb, or indeed harvesting a fruit or vegetable, take a moment of quietness to give the plant your full attention; then ask permission in simple, everyday terms: "Is it OK if I take some of what you have to offer?" Practise becoming receptive to the response. Most of the time this is going to be a quiet sense of acquiescence, a knowing that you have the requested permission. Occasionally there might be a counter question, requesting perhaps your commitment to the highest ethical standards. Reassure the plant that you have their best interests at heart and are working for the benefit of all sentient beings and then make an offering—it might be an emotional offering of simple gratitude. Or perhaps you might be guided to gift the plant something physical—an amulet or charm, or even food.

However you visualise this, the adoption of an attitude of respect and mutual co-operation is vital if your relationships are going to develop in useful and meaningful ways. One of the main contentions of this book, which we will explore more thoroughly in the final chapter, is that developing our relationships with plants in ethical co-creation and conscious co-dependency is a highway to emotional maturity and full ecological responsibility.

Using a pendulum

Some practitioners advocate the use of a pendulum, and I myself have used—and still use—this method of verifying responses. Pendulum users will tell you that the method is simply a way of tuning in to your own intuition, to use a contemporary analogy. Like any other method, however, you need to practise it and become familiar with your own energy dynamics. Once mastered, the pendulum can be a valuable tool for communication, although increasingly I find these days I no longer need it. One gets better, over time, at moving directly to the place of knowing.

A simple guide to using the pendulum, however, might look like this. First, choose a pendulum that has some meaning, significance or attraction for you. Preferably it will be made from natural materials—wood, stone or crystal. Handle your pendulum frequently, so that it may absorb your specific personal frequency. Use it for simple questions when you have a decision to make or simply need some guidance on any matter. It is important, however, to remember that you are not obliged to obey it: that is not the point. You are merely gathering information.

The first thing to do is establish the directions of swing for the values of "yes" and "no". My personal pendulum rotates clockwise for yes and anticlockwise for no, but others tell me it is the other way around for them, or that it is a simple back and forth swing versus a side-to-side swing. To check what yours wants to do, simply hold it suspended and ask a question to which you already know the answer—such as, "Is my name Peter?" Observe the pendulum start to move and note its direction. Then ask it a question whose answer you know to be false, for example, "Is my name Amanda?" Again, note the direction, which should be a distinct counterpoint to the "yes" direction.

Having established this, you can proceed to "talking" to a plant. The plant can be there or not: perhaps at first it will be helpful to have it physically present, but the plant essence or spirit can be contacted even if it is not physically present. I usually start with, "Am I in communication with the spirit of [insert name of plant]?" If I get a yes to this, I then ask, "Are you willing and able to help me with [nature of the problem]?" This is the preamble to asking for the guidance you need, but remember, questions will need to be framed so that they may be answered as either "yes" or "no". There's no point in asking, for example, "What do you expect me to do about such-and-such a problem?" as this cannot be answered with a simple yes or no.

Once you have made progress in understanding how individual plants may help—for example, wormwood, and *Artemisia* species generally, are extremely effective at dealing with parasitic influences, nettle's energy is protective, and so on—you can ask for help in resolving specific issues. Simply ask the plant to signal willingness to help, then check that the help has been given, and finally offer the plant your grateful thanks and relax confident in the knowledge that your request has been answered. There is only one caution: do not use these techniques to try to harm or disadvantage any other being: plants, as we saw in Chapter 7, are fully aware of intention to harm, and you may find that your supplication renders you vulnerable to being taught a karmic lesson—which will be in your best interest, in the fulness of time, but which you may not welcome in the short term.

As I have indicated throughout this book, I have given illustrative examples of the nature and effects of a few plants, but it is not my intention here to provide a definitive list of such actions. Partly this is because it can be a highly individual matter, and the relationship a plant has with you may be very different from that it has with anyone else. As an example, when I first journeyed (see below) to meet wormwood, she presented herself to me as a grey-haired, bespectacled academic wearing a red cardigan and a beige tweed skirt, with stockings and sensible shoes into the bargain, sitting in a library. Most experience her as a quintessential witch. I was completely convinced by her contemporary choice of avatar, however, and the message she gave was authentic and to the point.

Do remember, however, that these beings will have real and compelling personalities, and as such they may be unpredictable, ungovernable, mischievous, wise, playful, teasing, and occasionally narcissistic, pompous or facetious. These latter qualities, however, may actually reflect portions of your own personality, so do not be too quick to judge or criticise.

Journeying with plants

One of the best ways to get to meet your plant allies "in person" is through the shamanic practice of journeying. Usually there is preparation for this involving the ingestion of the plant as a tea, tincture or essence (similar to a Bach Flower or Australian Bush Remedy), but it is advisable to be able to taste the plant, so preferably not in capsule form. The journey is best conducted by an experienced leader, guide or storyteller, possibly accompanied by a simple, repetitive drum beat, and generally starts with an eyes-closed relaxation and visualisation.

From a specific and descriptive starting point, which you are invited to flesh out in your own imagination, the guide will then draw you into the journey by suggesting a path or a trail to follow, leading to another specific location, in which you will encounter the spirit of the plant. You will be given the instruction to note the appearance of the plant-person, its gender, physical characteristics and clothing, and to give free rein to your own imagination in fleshing out the appearance of this personage, again, without self-censorship or judgment. Then you will be invited either to receive a gift, or a teaching from the plant. Listen and receive in gratitude, and if invited, hold a longer conversation with the personage, until invited to visualise the plant-person withdrawing, and following your own path back to the starting point, before gently awakening to your mundane reality.

I have described one of my own journeys at the start of Chapter 7, with the spirit of hawthorn, and I give a brief description of another journey I took with horsetail below. You will note the appearance of gender as a descriptor in these fantasies (and by the way, I am not using the word fantasy in a pejorative sense). The gendering of plants is second nature and familiar in cultures who embrace these practices, as Stephen Harris and Françoise Freedman extensively discussed in their essay, *Shamanic Plants and Gender in the Healing Forest*.[7] As one Master Curandero from Tarapoto in Peru reports, speaking of tobacco, "I have seen him … The father of tobacco is a strong, tall, black man … he wears a white hat and his eyes shine like fire, but he is good, he takes care of us."[8]

When it comes to debates about the gender of specific plants, and without getting involved in botanically complex and convoluted explanations, I find it best to exercise tolerance and permissiveness. It has a lot to do with the individual seeker. If you journey with a plant and that plant appears to you as a woman, then for you it does indeed adopt a female persona. End of. It is not something that can be independently verified, as all such encounters are necessarily and intensely subjective. My advice is always to accept what is given to you in your vision, and if you don't always understand it, simply make comprehensive notes (every journey should be followed with a quiet period for noting down one's experiences) and review them at a later date, when perhaps your ongoing experience will be able to help in decoding the message.

By all means find out what other practitioners and writers have discovered about communicating with plants. One of my favourite books on the subject is Pam Montgomery's *Plant Spirit Healing*.[9] Another favourite writer on these matters is Stephen Harrod Buhner, especially *The Secret Teachings of Plants*[10] and *Plant Intelligence and the Imaginal Realm*.[11] I have not sought to re-present the work of these seminal authors, preferring to develop my own insights and methods, but they have been constitutional in my own journey of discovery, and so I recommend them to your attention. Both these authors offer practical instruction in relating to, and communicating with, plants. My strong suggestion is that you take it upon yourself to research and develop your own methods, and your own relationships. They will be among the most rewarding that you can find in this world.

One of Pam's ideas, which I have already referred to, was immediately intuitive for me when I heard her lecture at one of the Plant Consciousness events, and that was the suggestion that we do not need to ingest the plant in order to receive its benefits, nor even be in close proximity to it. We can call upon the plant at any time, knowing its character to embody the particular energy that you need in the moment. For example, if you suspect or know that you are surrounded by what might be described as a parasitic energy or influence, you might call upon wormwood without ceremony to assist you in clearing it from your physical, emotional and energetic fields on an acute basis. This is always done "for the greater good of all" and without intention of harm to any being. You can feel the protection pretty much immediately. Imagination, some will say. Well, remember what I have been saying about imagination! Placebo, as even scientists are apt to comment, is a powerful principle.

With this approach, the sky is the limit—or should that be the cosmos?—when it comes to what you may achieve. You will, however, need to research and get to know your plants by any and all means possible, including academic research and personal encounter. You will, if nothing else, dramatically increase your circle of friends.

* * *

I crossed a wide prairie, making my way towards a bank of trees in the distance. As I grew nearer, I saw a gap in the trees and slightly altered my course to join the forest at that point, thinking it to be the issue of some path or trail into the interior. Instead, when I arrived, I immediately understood that this was where I needed to be to meet the spirit of horsetail—*Equisetum arvense* (meaning horsetail of the meadow), who frequently likes to grow close to the banks of streams. Looking around the immediate area, I saw the stream, gushing out of the forest and playfully tumbling into and across the meadow. I laid myself down by the stream and relaxed, lulled into a hypnogogic state by the babbling of the water.

Horsetail came to me in this reverie as an American Indian warrior, dressed in a magnificent headdress of rainbow feathers. However, on looking closely I saw that these were not in fact feathers at all, but brilliantly luminescent fronds of horsetail herb, glowing with an intense inner light. I explained that I wanted to know more about his healing actions, as I felt I had been called by him to make more use of his abilities in my practice. He gave me one very simple message. I say simple, but it has taken me 3 or 4 years to fully decode it, and I still continue to draw significance from it. He said, "I become what I want to destroy."

Horsetail is known in herbal medicine as a urinary astringent, in which context it is second to none. In my mind, it had already signalled that it might fulfil many of the requirements of a *qi tonic*, in TCM, helping to build strength and vitality in the body, as well as preventing the loss of fluids. In the German tradition there are reports of its potency as an anti-cancer herb. The plant is known for its high content of silicon, and as a homeopathic and tissue salt remedy, silica is used to remove foreign objects, especially metals, from the body. I have since ascertained that the plant can assist in counteracting the ill effects of too much silicon in our environments, with the obvious connotation of silicon chips and the computer-dependent "solutions" to which, as a race, we are in process of becoming dangerously addicted.

Horsetail holds a place in my inner circle of plant allies.

Notes

1. Roberts, J. (1970). *The Early Class Sessions*, Book 2: ESP Session January 13, 1970, p.10
2. Lodwick, L. (2014). *Evergreen Plants in Roman Britain and Beyond: Movement, Meaning and Materiality. Cambridge University Press online.* Available at: https://www.cambridge.org/core/journals/britannia/article/abs/evergreen-plants-in-roman-britain-and-beyond-movement-meaning-and-materiality/652BA73F006FBEE701FF00529FA746AC. Accessed 28.12.25.
3. Taylor, K. (2009). Biological Flora of the British Isles: *Urtica dioica* L. *Journal of Ecology, 97*: 1436–1458. https://doi.org/10.1111/j.1365-2745.2009.01575.x.
4. The College of Naturopathic Medicine: https://www.naturopathy-uk.com/product/herbs_for_everyday_living/.
5. Coleridge, S. T. (1834). *Biographia Literaria: Or, Biographical Sketches of My Literary Life and Opinions*. New York: Leavitt, Lord & Company, p. 175.
6. Roberts, J. (1995). *The Magical Approach: Seth Speaks about the Art of Creative Living*. San Francisco: Amber Allen Publishing.
7. Harris, S. & Freedman, F. B. (2010). Shamanic Plants and Gender in the Healing Forest. In *Plants, Health and Healing: On the Interface of Ethnobotany and Medical Anthropology*, ed. Elisabeth Hsu and Stephen Harris. New York: Berghahn Books, pp. 135–178. https://doi.org/10.1515/9781845458218-008.
8. Mabit, J. & Giove, R. (2012). *Sinchi, Sinchi, Negrito: Medicinal Use of Tobacco in the Upper Peruvian Amazon*. Available at: https://www.takiwasi.com/docs/arti_ing/sinchi_sinchi_ing.pdf. Accessed 24.12.2025.
9. Montgomery, P. (2008). *Plant Spirit Healing: A Guide to Working with Plant Consciousness*. Rochester, VT: Bear & Company.

10. Buhner, S. H. (2004). *The Secret Teachings of Plants: The Intelligence of the Heart in the Direct Perception of Nature*. Rochester, VT: Bear and Company.
11. Buhner, S. H. (2014). *Plant Intelligence and the Imaginal Realm: Into the Dreaming of Earth*. Rochester, VT: Bear and Company.

CHAPTER TEN

Return of the light: the medicine of the human

Come as you are, as you were
As I want you to be
As a friend, as a friend
As an old enemy.

Kurt Cobain[1]

Known as the Big Freeze of '63, the winter of 1962 through 1963 goes down in history as one of the most extreme in modern times in the British Isles. Despite that, and despite snowfall on either side of the day itself, it did not qualify as a White Christmas.

On Christmas Eve of 1962 I travelled with my family—mother, father, two brothers and one very new sister—once more to *Elfins*, in the depths of Sussex, to spend the holiday with my maternal grandparents. I was fortunate, growing up, to have, and spend time with, both sets of grandparents, and I loved them both. We would typically spend every alternate Christmas, one year in Sussex, the next in London, or later Hertfordshire. Later still, when my parents moved to a bigger house, the grandparents started coming to us.

This year it was Sussex. Excitement ran high, as usual, and getting to sleep was almost impossible. Christmas was, well, Christmas, a lazy day of presents, food and fun, entertained by my grandfather's magic tricks, and fed by the bounty of my grandmother's ample kitchen table. Late on Boxing Day it began to snow—although we were in bed by then and did not discover it until the next morning. It was a mere inch or two, nothing much in comparison with what was to come, but enough to make some snowballs and a small snowman. Then again, late on 29 December (the day before my grandmother's birthday), it began to snow again.

On the morning of 30th I woke up to something of a commotion. Running from the bedroom I was incredulous at what I saw. My father had opened the front door and was standing staring at a white wall that reached up to the top of the door frame, and quite possibly beyond. It took a moment to comprehend what was happening. Snowed in—completely, utterly. We checked the back door, and all the windows. It was the same. The small cottage was pretty much buried in a huge snowdrift. The back of the house was not quite as completely blocked—the blizzard had obviously been driving the snow up to the front elevation—and my father and grandfather went about the business of digging through from the kitchen door to the path surrounding the cottage and then attempting to make progress circumnavigating to the front door. A little later, having toiled relentlessly for a couple of hours, they knocked triumphantly on the front door, having cleared the bulk of the drift from the doorstep, and my grandmother let them in.

To us as kids this was THE single most exciting thing that had happened to us—probably ever. To my father however, we quickly realised, it was the source of some anxiety. He was due back in work on 2nd January. I can dimly remember the women trying to persuade him that it wasn't worth it. The roads were all blocked. There was no transport. Television footage, presumably taken from a helicopter, showed an almost uninterrupted white blanket across the whole of Southern England. He was adamant. Looking back, he reminds me of myself. Never one to let a small cataclysm get in the way of business. The adults hoped against hope that a thaw would happen by then, but everyone knew it wasn't likely—and if it did that the next thing we'd have needed to contend with was flooding—not a great improvement on being frozen in.

January 2nd arrived, and although there had been no appreciable increase in the volume of snow on the ground, neither had there been any sign of thaw. A telephone call to the railway company established that a limited service was running from Pulborough, and after confirming the times of departure my father resolved to walk to the station—a distance of just over 3 miles. Even if our car could have been excavated from its icy tomb and persuaded to start, the roads were still pretty much impassable to motor vehicles, even over that relatively short distance.

I remember us all huddling with my mother on the road watching his heavily over-coated figure disappear slowly through the drifts and the blizzard that was even now beginning to whip up again, dramatically wondering whether we'd ever see him again. Had I been a little older (I was 7) I might have captured echoes of Captain Lawrence Oates valiantly walking out into the Antarctic blizzard during the *Terra Nova* expedition of 1912, uttering the immortal words, "I may be some time". My father, however, arrived home safely and in time to go to work the next day, and as soon as the roads were somewhat clear, about two bliss-filled, school-free weeks later, he came to collect us.

The thaw was slow, which was a blessing in one way, in that floods were avoided. It was well into March before the last of the snow disappeared. In the weeks that followed I remember seeing the Thames near Richmond and Kew frozen so thick that it was declared safe for ice skaters—something that was rarely, if at all, seen since the 1800s, and which certainly hasn't happened since.

I also remember, because it was such a welcome contrast come late February, the emergence of the first green shoots appearing. The world awoke slowly, as if from a deep sleep, heralded by preternatural Spring shades of fresh green, hope and anticipation bursting from every bud. In some way I think I have been trying to retrieve that magic for a long time.

My drift—if you'll excuse the pun—is this. The depth of winter is ripe for hibernation, a break from all the busyness of the preceding months, and an opportunity to reflect and reset. At least that's how it can be, if we make appropriate plans. There is something intrinsically Northern about this, and the festival that we know as Christmas, despite its annexation to an altogether different spiritual tradition, owes its true familiarity and meaning to the old spirituality of the North. Evergreen Nordic trees and snow are not native to the Holy Land, needless to say.

There is a contemporary neo-pagan idea, which seems to be unrelated to any academically verifiable historical data, that the festival of Yuletide begins at the solstice on 21 December and lasts till 24th, followed by the Return of the Light on 25th. The word "solstice" comes from the Latin *sol* (sun) and *sistere* (to stand still), so named because at that point the sun appears to stand still before reversing and climbing higher into the sky again. This apparent standstill, it is said, is responsible for the 4-day interval that is devoted to the festival. Astronomically speaking there is a window of about 48 hours in which the solstice may in fact fall, and of course in itself it is only a moment—the actual point when the sun is at its lowest elevation—December in the Northern hemisphere, June in the Southern. And of course, the other way around for the summer solstice, when the sun is at the highest elevation.

It is easy to see how the Return of the Light could be an analogue for the birth of Christ, but the calendars are confused. In Germanic lore, where Yuletide originated, the festival lasts 12 days—as indeed reflected in the current customary 12 days of Christmas. At that era, however, the Winter Solstice was thought to fall on the 25th, but since the introduction of the Gregorian calendar it has been set as the 21st.

I personally like the idea of the 4-day intermission from 21 to 24 December, and over the last few years I have resolved to complete my business for the year by 20th at the latest, and then effectively to go on retreat. Those four days are sacrosanct, an opportunity to cut loose from onerous obligations and give my own trajectory some serious contemplation, giving thanks for the blessings of the year, and setting intentions for what is to come. Christmas itself then indeed becomes the Return of the Light—whether you prefer to see that as the arrival of Jesus of Nazareth among us, or whether you prefer to honour the chthonic gods of the North and the seasons and cycles of the earth itself.

Any which way, and not exclusively focusing on the deep cold winters of my childhood, over the last 60-odd years we have witnessed the erosion of sacred time in this season. Not merely by means of the manic run up to the festival, focused on the preparation for family visits and celebratory comestibles, as also upon the acquisition of material goods, and the sales (they used to be the "January" sales, which then started coming on Boxing Day, and are now pre-empted by "Black Friday" 4 weeks before Christmas, which is in fact an American invention related to Thanksgiving), but also the general feeling of unwillingness to interrupt the grindstones of business, commerce and industry for any meaningful length of time, the frenzied imperative to remain at all times productive and generate profit.

Whether or not you regard this as the deliberate colonisation that characterises capitalist ideology, inflicted upon us from above by our corporate masters and driven by low wages and high taxation, or whether you take the view that it is the sickness of our increased alienation from the natural world, and hence from the sacred, willingly embraced by a population devoid of a spiritual compass, the result is the same: competitiveness and aggression; anxiety and depression; leading often to lethargy and paralysis, and frequently culminating in a self-flagellatory New Year's Resolution to do "better" in the coming year—which usually means intensifying the pressure to be someone else, someone that you are currently not.

For the past four years I have been consciously observing the eight pagan festivals, or Sabbats, of *Imbolc, Ostara, Beltane, Litha, Lughnasa* (or *Lammas*), *Mabon*, *Samhain* and *Yule*. They are aligned to the summer and winter solstices and the March and September equinoxes, interspersed by the intermediate points in an eight-fold division of the solar year. (As a side note here, the Christian ecclesiastical calendar, after several confusing historical changes, has somewhat fudged the issue, particularly in relation to *Ostara*—Easter—once but no longer aligned to the lunar cycles, which can vary year on year by almost a month, and is therefore frequently disconnected from the true sabbat). *Litha*, the summer solstice, is similarly a 4-day event for us, and as it occurs very close to my own birthday, I regard it as a natural and intuitive opportunity for a longer break. For each of these festivals certain plants offer themselves as signifiers—for midsummer, for example, St John's wort comes forward. But there is not just one plant per festival: we all know that at Yuletide there are several, including the Nordic pine, the yew (whose "womb-like space" is the epitome of the comforting hug of midwinter), the mistletoe, and the musically celebrated holly and ivy.

You can choose your own plants, too. What I am humbly suggesting here is that we work to activate a far closer relationship with the natural world, and thus with the Nature in ourselves. This is not something that needs to be externally imposed upon us—the grudging allowance of a little breathing space every so often so we don't get too tired to function as the engines of endless—and mindless—production. The pattern is innate, the very flesh and habit of the reality that we occupy in time and space, the entirely natural and cosmological transit points that mark out the passage of our collective annual orbit of the sun, and therefore a deep and intimate part of each of us as earthly beings. It takes very little to start: merely add those dates, those festivals, to your private calendar, and resolve to give the matter just a few moments of your attention at the relevant seasons, to find out more about each one (bless the internet for easily accessed research options) and gradually infuse these ideas into your daily lives, if you are not already doing so.

* * *

Ethics are complex in our era. We are easily led by the many narratives that are presented to our bewildered and overtaxed eyes and ears, and of all the skills that we have developed over the aeons as a species, the art of selling things to each other—including perspectives, ideologies and opinions—is one of the most highly developed. So much so that we are now frequently completely and unflinchingly *convinced* about things of which we can have no personal in-depth knowledge or verification at all. Such issues may be political, legal, economic, ecological, charitable, medical, social, psychological, geographical, cosmological, and so on and on. We have opinions on everything, and we are keenly attentive to the opinions of others, which we use as indicators as to their approval rating—their basic worth, moral rectitude, and whether they are suitable people to associate with. But if we were to have to justify some of those opinions, we would rapidly find out three things: one, we don't know enough to be certain about any of them. Two, there are perfectly cogent arguments for almost any opinion that anyone may hold. Three, that, were we to ask ourselves how we formed, or where we obtained such an opinion, we might very well discover that someone had placed it there while we weren't looking.

In the end it comes down to what kind of person you are, or want to be, and whether you have enough humanity left to be able to activate basic compassion when it is called for—in whatever circumstance, including being able to embrace people who may have previously been excluded from your "approved" list. Stories of reconciliation, changes of heart, and the ability to forgive, to overlook differences and focus on common humanity, are the stuff of a thousand movies and stories that we avidly consume as "entertainment", while missing the object lesson, which is that we are being offered a mirror in which to view the distortions within our own hearts and minds.

Many years ago, I was privileged to attend a gathering of devotees of the teacher, Jiddu Krishnamurti. Thousands of people convened in the grounds of Brockwood Park in Hampshire to listen to the teachings of this man, who had distinguished himself by refusing to accept the mantle for which he had been groomed by his Theosophical guardians, that of the prophesied World Teacher. Krishnamurti had broken ranks with his promoters and followed his own ministry, strongly advising against following any doctrine, discipline, teacher, guru, or authority, including his own. On the occasion in question, he offered the observation that the way we define ourselves, for example via our national or religious identity, is a trap in which we limit ourselves and create divisions between ourselves and others. That evening in the campsite I had to listen to a close neighbour of ours reasoning that Krishnamurti couldn't possibly be referring to him and his immense pride in his Scottish heritage. Well at least he was following the exhortation not to follow the teaching—if you get my drift.

In terms of compassion teachings, one of my favourite meditations is the Buddhist *Metta Bhavana*—the loving-kindness meditation. This five-stage practice invites us to start by summoning love towards oneself; then for those close to us—friends and family perhaps; then moving on to neutral acquaintances; and then to someone you may actively dislike. Finally, the meditation is extended towards everyone equally—your community, your city, your country, and the whole world. However, my own Tibetan Buddhist teacher, Ato Rinpoche, offered a beautifully simple, but somewhat challenging definition of compassion when he suggested that, upon looking out onto your garden in winter, when snow and frost are thick upon the ground, offer the leftovers from your breakfast to the birds and animals struggling to survive. Note that he did not say, offer your breakfast itself, nor make a special provision. He said, rather than throw the unused food away, give it to someone who may need it. There is a simplicity of consideration here that does not override anyone's self-determination but is simply a benevolent acknowledgment of their right to exist.

Nature, we are told, is bountiful. There is enough for everyone. At least that is what they say. And then in the next breath we are cautioned with lack and poverty, and the fear of missing out. In Nature, if you watch, there is a natural order in the distribution of resources, including food. Individuals, of whatever species, are self-serving, first and foremost, but they do not overconsume, and when they have eaten their fill, they leave the residue to the next comer. It is a false modesty to deprive yourself while making a show of feeding others. Self-immolation does not militate towards survival. In a healthy community, every individual has their role, and therefore there is a need to respect the needs of every individual, while also recognising that every individual is different, and must follow their own path.

I might offer the opinion (of course it is just an opinion) that if humans were better behaved, we would not need charity. If financial, legal and political systems were not rigged to foster and protect the interests of a privileged elite, if care in the context of health and welfare were focused upon the interests of the end users rather than those of the industry and its shareholders, and if the resources of the natural world were regarded as the birthright of all, rather than opportunistic pickings for the few, then perhaps there would be less work for charitable enterprises. Instead, fuelled by the Darwinian misconception of "survival of the fittest" (which is not even an intelligent reading of Darwin), we license large-scale corporations to act as they see fit, even if it means the destruction of habitats, the impoverishment of marginal and unvalued communities, and the profligate depletion of vital reserves, while those who have benefited the most then reinvent themselves as "philanthropists" and invest their insanely overinflated fortunes in "good works" that somehow succeed in coming full-circle once more to increase their bulging coffers. (*Ker-ching.*)

I could offer the *opinion*, again, that emotional immaturity due to unconscious and unresolved post-traumatic stress disorder is the norm among humans. Where does this come from? What are the stressors, and how did they get there? The question is too large for this volume. A recent newcomer on the "save the world" platform is Australian biologist, Jeremy Griffith, whose analysis presented in his book, *Freedom: The End of the Human Condition*, suggests that a psychological conflict arose in early hominids when they started to develop *intellect*, and found themselves at odds with *instinct*, by which their lives had previously been guided.[2] The echo of the Genesis story of the Fall is not lost on commentators (or indeed on Griffith himself), but although the idea has merit—there is indeed a clash between instinct and, if not intellect, then at least some idea of autonomy governed by an ability to make decisions on the basis of reflection and analysis—there are also many unexamined assumptions about the degree and nature of "intelligence" among our supposed antecedents, the primates, or indeed any animal species.

I guess it's one of the big unanswered questions about human existence, which is not to say that we are unwise to try and discover the meaning behind it, but my main problem with all such explanations is that they leave out huge areas of our psychological and spiritual reality, and function only on a very restricted register of experience and theoretical perspective. Human nature, what humans are and do, how they frame and justify their actions, is a complex phenomenon, and probably few "evil" people actually believe they are evil—and that assessment probably extends to the most evil people the race has ever produced (think Hitler, Stalin, Vlad the Impaler, Pol Pot, or closer to home, Fred and Rosemary West, or Ian Brady and Myra Hindley). They may be psychopaths, of course, prone to antisocial behaviour and lack of empathy while apparently maintaining a high-functioning, "normal" exterior, but psychiatric categories are frequently found to be extremely difficult to measure and validate, and therefore to a large extent they resist the objective confirmation to which they aspire—and therefore frequently also the appropriate social response.

Then there is religion. Ostensibly developed to provide a much-needed moral compass, as well as some semblance of meaning in a world that can seem all too random and meaningless, religions are also rather prone to enacting agendas of prohibition, judgment and control, while frequently also functioning as smokescreens for the less desirable traits of those who promote them: narcissism, greed, concupiscence, cruelty and abuse—including child abuse. Religion, in the company of other manifestations of extremist ideology, is also frequently found to provide grounds for violent disagreement, brutal repression and war. The other side of religion, the conviction of the reality of personal salvation, peace, and meaning, would be just fine without the seeming necessity to convert all and sundry to one's own way of thinking, on pain either of exclusion from the community of souls, or eternal damnation.

Neither do I think it appropriate to retreat fully into forms of spirituality gleaned from prior epochs, or indigenous societies that we have long plundered for their lands, their natural wealth, and their human rights, and now, all too often, their assumed spiritual superiority (a two-edged compliment), their ceremonial allies, and their magical prowess. To experience the personal and intimate tuition available from the plants involved is one thing. The purpose of that is not to throw away one's one heritage and play at being "shamanic": it is to do the work of growing, and *growing up*, that being human demands—not only at this era of history, but throughout history, and over and over again, until we "get it". We learn from the plants how to be truly human, which is to say, we receive guidance as to the correct and appropriate response not to some imagined "condition" from which we suffer, but to the challenges that we face in our "ordinary" lives right now. I cannot put this too strongly. And it doesn't just apply to the powerful so-called Master Plants that we met in Chapter 7, but to all or any plants, as I hope I succeeded in promoting in Chapter 8.

Similarly, in invoking the pagan festivals, I am not advocating play-acting, pretending to be Druids and what not—although I am completely OK with the preservation of arcane knowledge of previous eras. In fact, I advocate it in preference to ditching the wisdom of our predecessors as somehow irrelevant and anachronistic. But specifically, I am suggesting a template for the restructuring of contemporary time according to the natural cycles of Earth, which every one of us is free to enact in our own lives, using our own calendar, in collaboration with the plants that surround us, and offering up our own unique sets of problems and challenges as the material to be worked with, and possibly transformed, resolved, or even redeemed—and I chose that word deliberately, not necessarily in the sense of an ultimate apotheosis, but in the sense of a voucher that you might redeem in exchange for something that you need or want. That is the magic that is available to all of us, the ability to transform, reimagine and recreate our lives using the very material that superficially appears to be "the problem".

In terms of emotional maturity—and actually I think most human problems arise from a mistaken conceptualisation of emotion, in that we are constantly blindsided by our inability to accept our emotions unconditionally—my previous book, *The Mind's Eye*, offers a perspective that can assist us to transform difficult emotions by understanding their true purpose, which is that of a teacher. What I am suggesting here, to supplement that, is that we can also call upon plants to assist with this. Whether we "take" (ingest) them to try and ease the pain of what we feel, or to enhance our understanding of the issue; whether we use them in more refined essences, such as the Bach repertoire, to directly address emotional stasis and impasse; or whether we adopt them as psychic allies for their individual personality, character and talents, welcoming plants into our lives as fully as we can is to invite vitality, hope, excitement and joy, as natural emotional counterparts of fatigue, despair, frustration and dejection.

A spiritual renaissance of our time is afoot. I cannot say whether it is any more or less potent or significant than any other similar event in history—I have no personal frame of reference or means of comparison.

I do know that I have been expecting it, that I received intimations of it early in life, and that "chance" literary encounters, especially during my twenties, seemed to confirm it. The *Seth* material by Jane Roberts, already referred to in previous chapters, was a significant part of this discovery, but antecedents can be found in the prophesies of Edgar Cayce (the Sleeping Prophet), and the writings of various members and associates of the Theosophical Society, such as Alice Bailey, among many others.

Before I came into contact with any of that, in 1979 I chanced upon a book called *The Six o'Clock Bus*, by Moira Timms.[3] The book presented an overarching prophetic timeline of aeonic reach, from the *Yugas* of Hindu philosophy, the Book of Revelation, the Mayan prophesies, through to astronomical calculations of the immense cosmic cycle of the secession of the equinoxes, all of which seem to point to the present age as the realisation and enactment of a planned awakening of epic, not to say apocalyptic, proportions. My sense of excitement on reading this material was confirmatory. It was as if I knew and remembered in the deepest part of myself what I had come here for, and in various ways it has informed all my most life-defining decisions, including the decision to study and practise natural medicine, which I saw as the necessary combination of the wisdom of body, mind and spirit, coming to us from the most ancient portions of our collective history, and being reinvigorated in our time in a movement that is at once a renaissance and an act of resistance.

Once this was embedded into my trajectory, along came the plants. As I have signalled in some of the more personal stories in this book, they have always been there, waiting in the wings—as I believe that they are for all of us, not just me—and then as time went on becoming more insistent and illuminating in their teachings and their influence. In Chapters 4, 5 and 6 I have specifically attempted concise rationales for the use of plants as primary medicines for humans, and for what they can teach us about the true nature of healing. It is a complex and ever-evolving story. I believe that plants evolve and adapt their abilities and their skills just as we do, in response to the needs of the epoch, and of those with whom they interact in their environment.

As herbalists we often experience a shortfall or unavailability of a particular plant that we want to use. My advice to students in the clinical situation is to find another plant which may be substituted in its place. In an academic context this usually involves a search through the literature to find herbs with similar known actions, but I have occasionally been surprised when an ostensibly completely unrelated and unlikely plant presents itself. When this happens, I take a moment to check it out: "You mean you can do this?" "Yes, I can do it." "Well OK then. Let's do it." Often, when checking this out afterwards I am able to validate it by reference to some corner of the literature, or to an alternate cultural tradition or geographical usage that I had not previously been aware of. In other words, the usage was known, although not to me or within my native tradition, and the plant itself had communicated this fact to me. On that basis, more often than not, I trust the information I am getting before checking, and of course my knowledge of plant medicine is sufficiently developed to avoid any possible pitfalls in terms of adverse effects and safety considerations.

Are we humans capable of similar willingness and flexibility? Are we willing to offer our medicine to the world? Are we able to trust that we have the required qualities and the creativity to bring to the table in response to the extraordinary needs of this epoch? Are we prepared to do the legwork of self-development in preparation for what the world might demand of us, individually? And are we able to accept that our difficulties have been given to us for a reason that might extend towards problem-solving for the world at large, and are not merely a personal battle with our demons?

In natural healing we recognise the existence of a universal healing energy that we call the *vis medicatrix naturae*—the healing power of nature. This healing power is nothing more or less than our own essential nature, our inner essence and light, which through the various techniques and modalities of natural medicine we can recruit to heal ourselves from within. But it is also the energy that we call upon to make deep transformational changes in any area of life, and it is our birthright. It belongs to us, and in itself it costs nothing. The only thing remaining to be discovered is how to activate it.

Bruce Lipton talks about our bodies as a receiver of a unique signal that is us, each of us individually.[4] He says that our very cells are tuned to this frequency, and are constantly receiving the signal, which literally keeps us alive from moment to moment. Remember the biblical saying, "Man shall not live by bread alone, but by every word that proceeds from the mouth of God".[5] This teaching from the temptation of Christ in the wilderness is the epitome of the idea. But we need to be open to receive it.

Susannah and Ya'acov Darling Khan, the founders of the School of Movement Medicine, also talk about *receiving* ourselves, specifically through awakening the dancer within and allowing that to be moved and animated by our essence. They also begin each session with an invitation to arrive at the practice exactly as we are in that moment, without judgment or self-criticism, as the prelude to discovering "the joy of knowing who you are and the fulfilment of making your unique contribution".[6] I have gained much from this teaching, coming into my life again as it did at a critical point in the writing of this manuscript.

When we do this, when we *receive ourselves*, we allow ourselves to become an antenna to the universe, through which our true nature can flow unimpeded, thus truly anchoring the light of the inner dimensions onto the Earth, and into the physical. Which is exactly what our plant brothers and sisters are already doing.

* * *

I awake in the very early hours of 3 January 2026 to find the room bathed in preternatural silver light. I throw open the window to view the eerie splendour of the full moon. The January moon is known as the Wolf Moon, and is, besides, a "supermoon", unusually large and bright. This year its appearance in my natal constellation of Gemini is all the more potent for me personally, as that is also its position in my natal chart.

My paternal grandmother used to warn me against viewing the full moon through glass, and although I laughed at her superstition at the time, something in me always remembers and heeds this advice. I'm not sure why. You never know what arcane wisdom may hide within these seemingly naive beliefs. Accordingly, I throw on a warm overcoat (it's something minus zero out there and I need to shut the window for everyone else's sake) and head out into the garden for some moon-bathing. It's crisp and cold, and a deep frost is in process. It is everything a deep winter's night should be, and yet it also holds the promise of brighter things to come.

The Wolf moon gets its name from North American native tradition and is so called because the biting frost of January makes food scarce in the wild, drawing wolves closer to human settlements in the hope of finding something. The spiritual connotations are endurance through hardship, introspection, and the releasing of old habits, but also warmth and comfort in the midst of deep cold. This year it appears with a similarly bright companion, Jupiter, easily seen as the two most powerful objects in the sky. Astrology does not currently feature among my core skills—although I did once study it—but I find on a quick search that a moon–Jupiter conjunction is associated with emotional warmth, generosity, wellbeing, optimism and belief in the good. I'll take that as auspicious for the conclusion of this manuscript.

It also occurs to me that there is another natural calendrical template in addition to the solar transits: that of the thirteen annual moons and their shifting cycles, which at 28 days per cycle add up to 364 days—one short of a full year, giving us the 365th "day out of time", according to the Mayan 13-moons calendar. The day out of time is an opportunity for a brief pause and reset, but it is also (some say) a portal, through which you can choose, if you wish, to walk into another timeline. That is to say, we can choose to activate the best world we can visualise, rather than stay with the old patterns that no longer serve.

Building on this, some say again, that the true meaning of the New Age concept of "New Earth", referred to in Moira Timm's book, the earth that we are told we may inherit if we are sufficiently developed and adequately prepared, is the mass choice of individuals to walk away from the old paradigm of fear, deprivation, lack, control, mistrust, exploitation, and the smoke and mirrors thrown up by the agents of misrule, and towards a new understanding of our role and place here on earth, manifesting instead joy, kindness, compassion, healing, communication, creativity, art and community with all beings.

Some talk of a "critical mass" needed to effect social and political change, and estimates vary between 5% and 25% in terms of what this may mean in hard numbers. Whatever the number, the one thing that stands out as critically important is that individuals take their role and their power seriously and vote with their feet for the things they prefer—which is another way of saying, walk through that portal to a better world. Your vote counts anyway, whether you exercise it consciously or not. Better to weigh in on the side of joy, compassion and exuberance; to emulate, perhaps, the ever-giving vitality and perennial endurance of plants, than remain stuck as victims of a psychology orientated towards and generated by fear and trauma.

When we plant a garden, be it for our own enjoyment, our own healing, or our own nourishment, or all the above, we consciously foster, protect and nurture the earthly life cycles of the plant beings, and they will repay us a thousandfold for doing so. Imagine the compressed power within a tiny seed, which through germination or propagation replicates itself over and over, endlessly giving its benefits to us, asking no more than that we respect, honour and celebrate its presence and its contribution to our lives.

I had a vision in which humans on the planet are indeed as the grass. But grass is remarkably tough and enduring. We play rugby and football upon it, and it endures. It forms the sward of our parks and meadows upon which children and adults play and relax. And it may indeed wither and die, as the passage from Isaiah that forms the libretto of the Brahms' Requiem has it. But it comes back. Again and again.

We cannot doubt our own place upon Earth. We cannot say that the Earth would be better off without us, without succumbing to the narrative of the orphan, the reprobate, the malcontent, the forlorn, the reviled, the destitute and the abandoned. The truth is we are always and forever connected to the Light. And if, as human grass, we also learn continually to "receive" the essence of ourselves, the light that we truly are, then our presence also benefits all life on Earth, and the human itself is restored to grace and health. As a friend of mine once put it, "All that is left of an arsehole once you burn the shit out of it is a divine being". And shit itself, as plants know well, is a magnificent fertiliser.

So be gentle with yourselves; honour and celebrate your individuality, your desires and preferences, and your cherished goals in life. These things are all part of your personal, individual medicine, and it is needed. And when narratives of deprivation, disenfranchisement and disenchantment threaten to take over, ask for a plant ally to enter your field, and be open to whoever answers that call.

Notes

1. Cobain, K. (1992). Come as you are. From *Nevermind* by Nirvana. DGC Records.
2. Griffith, J. (2016). *Freedom: The End of the Human Condition*. Sydney: WTM Publishing & Communications.
3. Timms, M. (1979). *The Six o'Clock Bus: A Guide to Armageddon and the New Age*. New York: HarperCollins.
4. Lipton, B. (2015). *The Biology of Belief: Unleashing the Power of Consciousness*. London: Hay House.
5. King James Bible, Matthew 4:4.
6. https://schoolofmovementmedicine.com.

EPILOGUE

Self-doubt is intuitive at some level. It demands that we constantly monitor our motives and our output, ostensibly to ensure that we are entirely congruent with our own highest values. That, as I would frame it, is its evolutionary purpose. But it can also undermine and paralyse. An argument that focuses, as this one does, on the ethics of human transactions in the natural world, risks invoking theory that may well prove too hot—and too voluminous—to handle. I am acutely conscious of the potential failings of my thesis. I can almost hear the objections, because, in another scenario, they are the objections that I myself might raise.

In fact, the business of writing is somewhat of that character—it's like having an argument with yourself. It consists in bashing the pro's and con's around to the nth degree, hoping that at some point the dust will settle to reveal the hidden gold, while all the while doubting whether the gold is in fact real, or merely fool's gold. In the end one must commit, for better or worse.

A former schoolteacher of mine was fond of saying, you don't have to provide an answer for everything. He was talking of a scenario in which one might offer a critique of, say, a political or ideological position, but offer no counter position, no solution to the problem that the original was attempting to solve. He likened it to taking away someone's cardiovascular disease and giving them cancer instead. I guess he didn't have too much faith in human problem-solving prowess—and probably with good reason.

In my private and my professional life, however, as those close to me will confirm, I am generally focused on solutions. I don't like to spend an hour or so discussing an issue and then not come up with some strategy that I think stands even an outside chance of success, or at least progress. So the question I am left with at the end of all this is this: have I delivered? Not just in terms of the persuasiveness of my argument, but in terms of what I have given the reader in exchange for the favour of buying and reading my book? And undoubtedly, partially at least, I tend to calibrate that in terms of practical benefit.

That is why I have devoted a chapter to giving practical tools with which to implement strategies of self-evidencing, by which I mean, I hope I have thrown down the gauntlet, at least, with regard to what my readers might do about all of this, if only in the privacy of their deepest, innermost meditations, and the restricted sphere of their own associates. That chapter stands out to my mind as different from much of the rest of the book, and that contrast is deliberate. Whether or not it works is for you to decide.

In the end, though, perhaps there are no answers. This continually self-creating, self-evolving symbol that we call reality, and into which we are each woven as the individual threads in some vast tapestry, is in itself an object of profound contemplation, and maybe we do not need to pathologise it at all. Maybe we just watch the show, enjoy the trip, go home to bed and hope it's all OK in the morning.

The one thing I dare to hope for is that you will find something to like, something to applaud, in these pages. Not because my ego is so fragile that I need the accolade—God knows I have been working alone on this for long enough not be dependent on anything so ephemeral as approval. But because, I guess in common with most people, I crave connection and confirmation. I am excited by the probability that there are others out there thinking the same way. Some may even have gotten "further" in the analysis and resolution of the various threads of concern that emerge in the discussion. I am eager to hear what you might add to the work, to the project.

If you are a fellow professional, I would hope that the elements that deal with that side of the arrangement between ourselves and plants have some merit in your own understanding of the project in which we are both engaged. I also hope that I have not destroyed too many sacred cows. I'm afraid it's a bit of a habit of mine.

To those who might complain that I am guilty of mixing and matching—and thereby possibly fudging—my ontological and epistemological perspectives, I would say simply this: it is time, if we are to solve these problems definitively, to cast our nets wide in search of ideas, from wherever they may come, and to forge bridges and connections with diverse schools of thought and expresssions of being, rather than reinforcing borders, fences and the delimitations of consciousness between species. It is time to admit that we are far more resourceful and creative than our current stultified cultural settings would have us believe. And it is time to recognise the intelligence, the creativity and the agency of all other organic and ensouled beings on our planet. It is time to step decisively into Planetary Citizenship.

From the Divine in Me to the Divine in You, in Sacred Time.

APPENDIX A

Comparative matrix: theories of plant consciousness

Dimension	*Conventional Science*	*Philosophical/Process Views*	*Ethnobotanical & Indigenous Perspectives*	*Esoteric & Channeled Teachings*
Core assumption about consciousness	Consciousness requires neural integration; plants behave intelligently but do not feel (Taiz et al., 2019).	Consciousness as process or field of experience (Whitehead, 1929; Varela & Maturana, 1980).	Consciousness is relational and distributed (Kohn, 2013; Viveiros de Castro, 1998).	All life is conscious; plants are ensouled or guided by group spirits (Blavatsky, 1888; Steiner, 1924; Roberts, 1972).
Key proponents/ sources	Trewavas (2003); Calvo (2017); Baluška & Mancuso (2009); Simard (2021).	Whitehead (1929); Marder (2013); Coccia (2018); Varela & Maturana (1980).	Kimmerer (2013); Schultes & Hofmann (1979); Davis (1996).	Theosophy; Steiner's Anthroposophy; Seth Material (Roberts, 1972); Ra Material (Elkins et al., 1984); Urantia Book (1955).
Nature of plant intelligence	Functional cognition: sensing, signaling, adaptive integration (Trewavas, 2017).	Plants 'think' non-representationally; world-making through growth (Marder, 2013).	Plants as teachers and kin; intelligence through relational communication (Kimmerer, 2013).	Subtle or etheric intelligences; communication with plant devas (Maclean, 1971; Buhner, 2004).
Evidence or method	Empirical: electrophysiology, Ca^2 signaling, GLR channels, root communication (Toyota et al., 2018).	Phenomenology, systems theory, panpsychist reasoning.	Visionary and ritual experience; ethnographic observation (Kohn, 2013).	Clairvoyant or channeled communication; direct inner perception (Steiner, 1924; Roberts, 1972).
Ethical/practical implications	Plant welfare considered ecologically; limited moral status (Taiz et al., 2019).	Ethics of participation and co-flourishing (Coccia, 2018).	Reciprocity and respect toward plant persons (Kimmerer, 2013).	Cooperation with devas or spirits; sacred cultivation (Steiner, 1924; Maclean, 1971).

Baluška, F. & Mancuso, S. (2009). *Signaling in Plants*. Springer.

Blavatsky, H. P. (1888). *The Secret Doctrine: The Synthesis of Science, Religion, and Philosophy*. The Theosophical Publishing Company.

Buhner, S. H. (2004). *The Secret Teachings of Plants: The Intelligence of the Heart in the Direct Perception of Nature.* Bear & Company.

Calvo, P. (2017). What Is It Like to be a Plant? *Journal of Consciousness Studies, 24*(9–10): 205–227.

Coccia, E. (2018). *The Life of Plants: A Metaphysics of Mixture*. Polity Press.

Davis, W. (1996). *One River: Explorations and Discoveries in the Amazon Rain Forest*. Simon & Schuster.

Elkins, D., Rueckert, C. & McCarty, J. (1984). *The Law of One: Book I (The Ra Material)*. Schiffer Publishing.

Kimmerer, R. W. (2013). *Braiding Sweetgrass: Indigenous Wisdom, Scientific Knowledge, and the Teachings of Plants*. Milkweed Editions.

Kohn, E. (2013). *How Forests Think: Toward an Anthropology Beyond the Human*. University of California Press.

Maclean, D. (1971). *To Hear the Angels Sing: An Odyssey of Co-creation with the Devas of Nature*. Findhorn Press.

Marder, M. (2013). *Plant-thinking: A Philosophy of Vegetal Life*. Columbia University Press.

Roberts, J. (1972). *The Seth Material*. Prentice-Hall.

Schultes, R. E. & Hofmann, A. (1979). *Plants of the Gods: Origins of Hallucinogenic Use*. McGraw-Hill.

Simard, S. (2021). *Finding the Mother Tree: Discovering the Wisdom of the Forest*. Alfred A. Knopf.

Steiner, R. (1924). *Spiritual Foundations for the Renewal of Agriculture (The Agriculture Course)*. Rudolf Steiner Press.

Taiz, L., et al. (2019). Plants Neither Possess Nor Require Consciousness. *Trends in Plant Science, 24*(8): 677–687.

Toyota, M., Spencer, D., SawainTodoriki, K. et al. (2018). Glutamate Triggers Long-distance, Calcium-based Plant Defense Signaling. *Science, 361*(6407): 1112–1115.

Trewavas, A. (2003). Aspects of Plant Intelligence. *Annals of Botany, 92*(1): 1–20.

Trewavas, A. (2017). *Plant Behaviour and Intelligence*. Oxford University Press.

The Urantia Book. (1955). Urantia Foundation.

Varela, F. J. & Maturana, H. R. (1980). *Autopoiesis and Cognition: The Realization of the Living*. D. Reidel.

Viveiros de Castro, E. (1998). Cosmological Deixis and Amerindian Perspectivism. *Journal of the Royal Anthropological Institute, 4*(3): 469–488.

Whitehead, A. N. (1929). *Process and Reality*. Macmillan.

www.ingramcontent.com/pod-product-compliance
Ingram Content Group UK Ltd.
Pitfield, Milton Keynes, MK11 3LW, UK
UKHW021938100926
8560IPUK00004B/46

9 781801 522489